From Memories to Mental Illness

A Conceptual Journey

EMOTIONS, PERSONALITY, AND PSYCHOTHERAPY

Series Editors:

Carroll E. Izard, *University of Delaware, Newark, Delaware*
and
Jerome L. Singer, *Yale University, New Haven, Connecticut*

Current volumes in the series

THE COGNITIVE FOUNDATIONS OF PERSONALITY TRAITS
Shulamith Kreitler and Hans Kreitler

FINDING MEANING IN DREAMS: A Quantitative Approach
G. William Domhoff

FROM MEMORIES TO MENTAL ILLNESS: A Conceptual Journey
William M. Hall

IMAGERY AND VISUAL EXPRESSION IN THERAPY
Vija Bergs Lusebrink

THE PSYCHOLOGY OF EMOTIONS
Carroll E. Izard

QUANTIFYING CONSCIOUSNESS: An Empirical Approach
Ronald J. Pekala

THE ROLE OF EMOTIONS IN SOCIAL AND PERSONALITY
DEVELOPMENT: History, Theory, and Research
Carol Magai and Susan H. McFadden

SAMPLING INNER EXPERIENCE IN DISTURBED AFFECT
Russell T. Hurlburt

SAMPLING NORMAL AND SCHIZOPHRENIC INNER EXPERIENCE
Russell T. Hurlburt

THE TRANSFORMED SELF: The Psychology of Religious Conversion
Chana Ullman

A Continuation Order Plan is available for this series. A continuation order will bring delivery of each new volume immediately upon publication. Volumes are billed only upon actual shipment. For further information please contact the publisher.

From Memories to Mental Illness

A Conceptual Journey

William M. Hall

Columbia Area Mental Health Center
Columbia, Tennessee

Plenum Press • *New York and London*

Library of Congress Cataloging-in-Publication Data

Hall, William M., M.D.
    From memories to mental illness : a conceptual journey / William
M. Hall.
        p.   cm. -- (Emotions, personality, and psychotherapy)
    Includes bibliographical references (p.   ) and index.
    ISBN 0-306-45244-8
    1. Memory disorders. 2. Memory. 3. Cognition disorders.
    4. Recollection (Psychology) 5. Human information processing.
    I. Title. II. Series.
BF376.H35 1996
616.89--dc20   96-25549
                                                         CIP

ISBN 0-306-45244-8

© 1996 Plenum Press, New York
A Division of Plenum Publishing Corporation
233 Spring Street, New York, N. Y. 10013

10 9 8 7 6 5 4 3 2 1

Printed in the United States of America

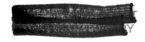

This volume is dedicated to the memory of my parents, Ruby and Bill, and to my wife and children for their love and support in this endeavor—Sara, Andrew, Fagan, and my beautiful new Laura "Bee."

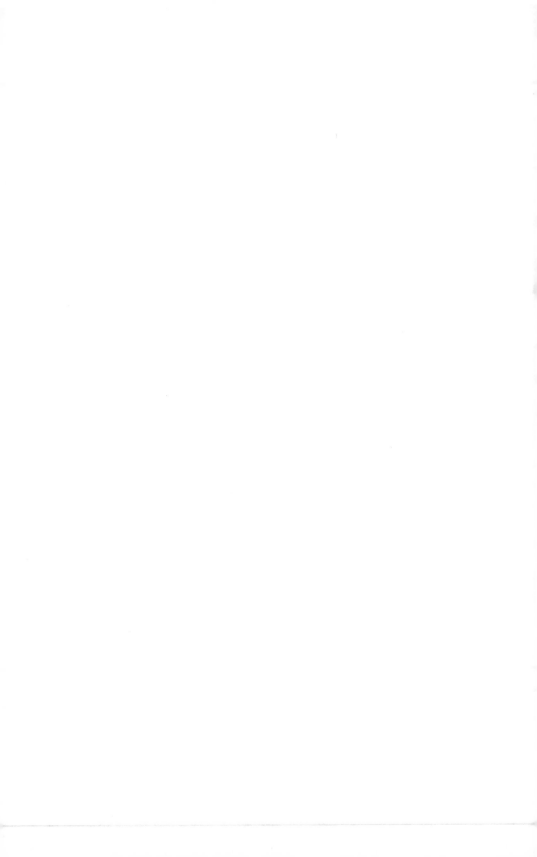

Preface

Perhaps the work presented here might best be described as a book of ideas. As the book's title implies, it represents a conceptual attempt to understand mental illness in relationship to such elemental brain processes as memory formation and storage. The journey begins with a consideration of some basic neural concepts. Through a pyramiding of related ideas, a theoretical framework that includes such sophisticated mental functions as thinking, consciousness, and the expression of emotion is developed. The ideas presented in this volume are consistent with the proposition that things that are associated in experience become physically linked as memories. As a consequence of this process, it is proposed that everything we learn is stored within the mind in associated fashion. Normal mental function is considered to arise as a direct consequence of this form of mental organization. Association seems to be the guiding influence that imposes order on what might otherwise be a system of cognitive and emotional chaos.

This volume is composed of two integrated parts. In the first part, an original hypothesis of the human brain is presented, based upon the ideas of association expressed earlier. Such an organizational arrangement may account for the associated nature of speech and thought, as well as the ability of one memory to stimulate the recall of similar memories. These ideas, in basic form, date back at least 300 years, to the writings of John Locke, and survive today as part of modern learning theory. The hypothesis presented represents an extension of these early ideas and deals with such concepts as specific and generalized memories, the function of emotion, the localization and retrieval of memories, the structure of consciousness, and the state-dependency of mood (Chapters 1–6).

By assuming that memories become electrically linked through associative experience, a biological basis for much of normal and pathological mental activity can be postulated.

In the second part of the book, the proposed hypothesis is used to provide a rational theoretical foundation for a number of psychiatric disorders (Chapters 7–9). In particular, such conditions as multiple personality disorder, psychogenic and organic amnesia, unipolar depression, and bipolar mood disorder are considered and interpreted from the perspective of this theory. Through this process, a unified biological basis for these psychiatric entities is developed, based upon the original hypothesis.

The theory presented here was not originally intended for publication. It was conceived as an attempt to integrate and better understand some of the complex psychopathology that I observed in patients. Initially, it consisted of a loose framework of ideas that arose from my curiosity about the associative nature of mental processes. Gradually, as older concepts were modified and new ideas were added, a coherent theory emerged. At the urging of friends and colleagues, I eventually committed it to paper for the purpose of publication. But the theory presented in these pages is by no means complete. As with any scientific hypothesis, the ideas that make it up should continue to evolve and undergo modification, as new facts about the brain are uncovered. I hope that this book will provide a useful framework for those who attempt to comprehend the human mind and mental illness.

Contents

Introduction

This volume is based upon the premise that associations between memories are basic to the very organization and function of the human brain. This single property may underlie our ability to think, reason, and memorize. By assuming memories are grouped in association as determined through experience, a functional and biological basis for most mental activity can be postulated.

For years, it has been recognized that many functions of the human brain seem related or associated in some way with each other. Such relationships that can be seen in virtually everything we do and think. Groups of ideas are strung together in sentences that follow each other in a logical, related sequence, suggesting they arise from an associated source. This phenomenon occurs so naturally that it generally goes unnoticed. When a failure in this natural linkage occurs, it becomes obvious and frequently is a sign of psychosis. If we look deeply into ourselves, we see that this basic associated organization is also present in our conscious thinking. Like the sentences that we utter, our thoughts flow in associated fashion from one related subject to the next. Memories trigger related memories, producing conscious thought and speech that are the outward manifestations of this associated organization. Sensory input from our environment triggers similar memories of past events that flash into consciousness. An idyllic country setting may produce the recall of a specific memory from our childhood, or a certain sound may bring back memories long since buried in our brains. Faces in a crowd may remind us of friends or associates. The smell of a certain perfume may trigger an emotional response associated with some special prior event. These are the obvious consequences of associated memory that

1

are familiar to us all. If we assume that memories are physically linked, as dictated by the naturally occurring relationships we observe, the associated nature of speech, thought, and other mental functions can be understood.

The observation that thoughts and memories are in some way associated is by no means new. Almost 300 years ago John Locke suggested that ideas exist in association with each other in the brain. Through the years this concept has continued to receive some support in one form or another. In *Briefer Psychology* (1890), William James conceptualized memories as existing in a framework of associations that stabilized them within the brain. In the 1970s, several investigators developed mathematical models for associative memories. These efforts became part of a larger attempt to create a new understanding of the brain by developing machines that mimic some aspects of human thought. The scientists who were engaged in this work became collectively known as *connectionists*. Their machines were termed *neural networks,* because they utilized multiple amplifiers linked in electronic circuits to simulate nerve cells connected by synaptic projections. Capacitors and resistors served to modulate current flow between amplifiers, simulating the variable ion flow that is thought to exist between neurons. Devices such as these have produced some remarkable results. Machines have been created that can solve large, complex problems without using the *brute force* technique of digital analog computers. Many of these devices seem to "learn" through experience, thus simulating biological function. Work in this area of artificial intelligence has expanded rapidly in the past 10 years and should eventually yield some important secrets of the brain. Some success has also been achieved at modeling systems composed of associative memories.

The work of connectionists is in part based upon a biological model for the brain proposed by Donald O. Hebb in 1949. In this work, Hebb suggested that memories exist in association because of specific modifications in the synaptic linkages that join them. When groupings of nerve cells are simultaneously activated, the synaptic linkages joining them become more conductive to neurotransmission. Associated memories are thus electrically linked more closely than unrelated memories. This assumption also plays an integral role in the hypothesis presented here.

By storing memories of our many activities in association, we maintain a mental record of their relationships as established through experience. An inner representation of the world is thus created, providing us with a standard by which all new data can be measured. This allows us to use the wisdom of prior experience to make literal and emotional interpretations of the things we encounter. It also functions as a natural filing system, enabling the rapid localization and retrieval of appropriate information. Associated memories seem critical to virtually every aspect of mental function. A disruption in this system may play a part in many types of mental illness. The hypothesis presented in these pages may provide new understanding for such mental conditions as depression, mania, multiple personality disorder, amnesia, and others.

As proposed in this work, associated memories are probably an essential part of the mechanism by which we think, reason, and understand the world. They seem to provide a reasonable physical explanation for the movement of thought among the neurons that constitute our memories. Even so, the concept of associated memory tells us little about the subjective composition and construction of thought. Why do we mentally dwell on certain issues and dismiss others as insignificant? Is there some reason thought flows in certain directions and not in others? It seems reasonable to assume that thought is not just a random movement of neurotransmission from one memory to the next. Some guiding influence must exist to give meaning and direction to this process. In this work, it is postulated that emotions serve this purpose. These entities are viewed as associations of memories that can be triggered as other related items. When memories are evaluated during thinking, the emotion released provides an interpretation that allows us to understand the significance and meaning of the issues under consideration. This information seems to motivate and determine the direction of subsequent thought. In effect, emotions are viewed as the main drivers of mental activity. The association of memories is thus felt to be the physical basis for the movement of thought, whereas emotional release is considered a major director of this process. It is further proposed in this work that some forms of mental illness result when memories and their emotional associations are mismatched. This effect may form the basis for minor distortions in thought as well as frank psychosis.

In this work, consciousness is viewed as an interface between the deeper reaches of the brain and the external world. Thinking is considered a cyclic process involving a stimulus–response mechanism. Stored memories can be recombined in consciousness to yield new thoughts with interpretations unique to their combination. Thoughts generated in this way can serve to stimulate additional thoughts perpetuating the cyclic process. Consciousness is thus regarded as a dynamic state in which stored memories can be mixed in various ways to produce new thoughts. In essence, consciousness is the *quality of mind* that allows us to think.

The reader should make no mistake about the intent of this work. Even though it is extensively referenced, it is not presented as a rigorous scientific theory based on a specific body of established research data. Such supporting documentation is simply not available at this time for many aspects of this work. Instead, it represents a hypothesis based upon the assumption that the brain is organized in associated fashion. It consists of a series of rational predictions and conceptualizations describing how such a system might function to produce normal and pathological mental activity. The greatest strength of this work may lie in its ability to conceptualize the human brain in a logical and coherent manner. The internal consistency of its ideas and ability to explain many functions of the human brain also suggest that it may have considerable scientific validity. Only time will determine if the general concepts presented will bear the burden of scientific proof and survive. At the very least, this work should provide an experimental framework for future thought and basic research.

The chief value of this work may lie in its ability to integrate established knowledge into a conceptual package that can be utilized directly in clinical and experimental applications. In most areas of science and medicine, this is generally accepted as a valid justification for the speculation that is inherent in theoretical work. In reference to a series of articles dealing with a theory of emotion (*affect theory*) that was recently published by *Psychiatric Annals,* the editor, Dr. Jan Fawcett (1993), illustrates this point by stating:

> While not always based on empirical data, this discussion of affect theory presents one very useful way of "bridging domains" as we struggle to integrate disparate levels of knowledge in formulating treatment strategies for our individual patients. While we certainly need as much empirical data as we can get and while this editor certainly subscribes to the edit that "one good experiment is worth a thousand expert opinions," in order to use the knowledge we have, to apply it most effectively for the benefit of our patients, we must have bridging concepts that allow us to integrate it. (p. 542)

This is exactly the philosophy and spirit that underlies the work presented here. It is hoped that the ideas contained in these pages will serve to *bridge gaps* in existing knowledge to allow a more comprehensive understanding of the human brain and mental illness.

General Considerations

It is proposed here that things that are associated in experience become physically linked as memories. Such an organizational arrangement would enable the brain to maintain in memory the many relationships it perceives in nature. As will be explained, this simple premise may underlie normal mental function and is central to the hypothesis presented

GENERAL OVERVIEW

In this chapter, some old concepts will be discussed and new ones introduced. In addition, enough anatomy and physiology of the brain will be included to provide adequate background support for the ideas considered. In subsequent chapters, additional concepts will be added and integrated into the overall theoretical framework. The hypothesis presented is a composite of many closely related and interwoven pieces.

The work presented in these pages represents a progression of related ideas that build upon each other in pyramiding fashion. Although the resulting hypothesis is quite abstract in places, an effort has been made to present it in a rational and coherent sequence. The general construction of this work was guided by the internal consistency of its many parts. In other words, an attempt was made at all levels to utilize only those elements that were compatible with other aspects of the overall hypothesis. There is admittedly much speculation involved but perhaps some real value also. The apparent strength of this work lies in its ability to explain many aspects of normal as well as pathological mental function, and to integrate them into a coherent whole.

The human brain is an exceedingly complex organ consisting of several cell types, collectively known as neurons. The communication of these cells with each other through the release of specific neurochemicals seems to form the basis for all mental activity. Microscopically, the brain appears to be a vast sea of such neurons interconnected by countless, thin, threadlike projections that facilitate this cellular communication. Some cells may be synaptically linked to literally thousands of other neurons, suggesting that many complex relationships exist. At each synaptic junction the flow of neurotransmission is transferred from one cell to the next by the release of specific molecules called neurotransmitters. Numerous such chemically distinct compounds have been identified, and many more probably exist. The flow of ions and neurotransmitters in the brain seems to form the basis for thought and all other functions of this organ.

HEBB'S POSTULATE

Our understanding of the brain has long been hindered by the extreme complexity of its microstructure. Even after years of research, we can only guess at the basic elements that encode memory. It is generally thought that a memory, or *engram*, is created in a cluster of neurons by specific modifications in the synaptic connections joining these cells. Either the amount or type of chemical transfer is presumably altered in a way that specifies the information contained in a memory. In effect, a discrete pattern of neurons representing a memory may somehow be created through these synaptic changes. Perhaps the information specifying a memory is dictated by the path of neurotransmission linking the neurons involved. In 1949, Hebb wrote in *The Organization of Behavior*: "When an axon of cell A is near enough to excite cell B or repeatedly or persistently takes part in firing it, some growth process or metabolic change takes place in one or both cells such that A's efficiency, as one of the cells firing B, is increased. (p. 62)" This might be explained by assuming that synaptic connections between neurons become stronger or more numerous when they are fired simultaneously. Presumably the flow of energy between such cells would be facilitated as a consequence of this increased electrical connectivity. Through these changes, neurons may somehow become grouped to reflect our perceptions of the world. This simple idea might form the basis for memory encoding.

Despite the wide acceptance of Hebb's ideas concerning synaptic plasticity, direct experimental proof was slow in coming. His ideas were eventually confirmed almost 25 years later by Bliss and colleagues (Bliss

& Garner-Medwin, 1973; Bliss & Lomo, 1973). These researchers found that brief bouts of electrical stimulation could strengthen the synaptic connections between rabbit hippocampal cells as measured by excitatory postsynaptic potentials. Hebb's original postulate has now been experimentally confirmed in a number of laboratories. In the following paragraphs, a mechanism for memory storage is outlined, based upon Hebb's original proposition.

SENSORY PERCEPTION AREAS

Within the brain are a number of specialized regions that receive and process data arising through sensory perception. These cortical structures are collectively known as *sensory perception areas*. At least one exists for each sensory modality. The visual cortex has been well characterized anatomically and is a good example of such a region. This structure is located in the posterior brain and receives intact images from the retina,

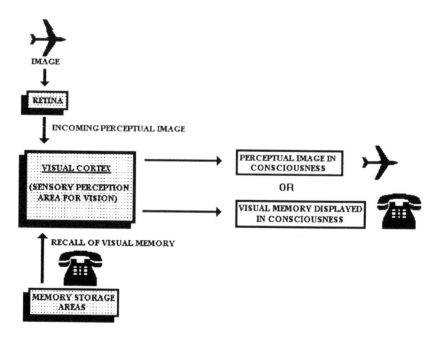

Figure 1.1 Images may enter consciousness from the recall of visual memories or by direct sensory perception, as illustrated here. The visual cortex represents the common pathway through which both entities pass. The telephone and airplane represent examples of common visual representations that can arise through sensory perception or memory recall.

which are then passed on to other brain regions for processing. Memory storage may start when information enters one or more of these specialized regions. Obviously much of the data processed here originates from direct sensory perception of the environment. It is proposed in this work that these structures may also process data arising from the recall of sensory memories. For example, a perception registered in the visual cortex may represent a current image recorded by the eyes, or may have arisen from the recall of a visual memory. In either case, the image would be displayed in consciousness because of its presence in this specialized cortical region. In a like manner, the auditory cortex might be stimulated by the sound of a friend's voice or simply by the memory of that voice. In fact, verbal thinking itself may largely arise from the recombination of auditory memories that are registered in this cortical region. The ideas presented here suggest that sensory perception areas function as *screens* upon which internal thoughts or external perceptions may be viewed in consciousness. This concept is illustrated in Figure 1.1.

STIMULATION OF SENSORY PERCEPTION AREAS DURING THOUGHT

It has long been known that the cortical perception areas play an active role in the uptake of new sensory data, but is there any evidence that these areas are also stimulated and utilized during normal thought, as predicted by this hypothesis? Such evidence would support the contention that these structures may function as screens upon which recalled memories can be displayed in consciousness. In 1977, Davidson and Schwartz used the technique of electroencephalography (EEG) to monitor brain electrical activity while subjects carried out visual and tactile imagery tasks. Alpha rhythm was simultaneously recorded for the brain regions associated with visual processes (occipital lobes) and tactile sensation (parietal lobes). It is known that alpha rhythm arising from a given brain region is suppressed when there is an increase in its activity. It was found that maximum suppression of alpha rhythm occurred in visual areas when subjects were involved in visual imagery. It was also determined that suppression was maximum in the parietal lobes when subjects were engaged in tactile tasks. These data suggest that the cortical perception areas may also be involved in the processing of data arising from the activation of memory during thought.

In a more recent study, Goldenberg, Steiner, Podreka, and Deeke (1992) measured the regional flow of blood to cortical areas when subjects answered questions that either did or did not require the use of visual imagery. This experimental technique is known as *regional cerebral blood flow* (rCBF) and involves the introduction and uptake of radioactive tracers, such as xenon-133, into the brain. Radiation is emitted in proportion to the amount taken up by a given region and is a measure of the local neural activity. In this study, it was found that regional blood flow varied greatly depending on the types of questions asked. When responses required the use of visual imagery, the occipital lobes became active. In contrast, challenges that required no imagery produced the opposite effect. Taken together, the EEG and rCBF studies suggest that the visual perception areas may also become active as a consequence of visual thought. This observation supports the concept that activated memory may reenter such regions in an attempt to duplicate the original sensory perception for the brain during the process of thought. Additional evidence in support of this idea is presented in later chapters.

FLOW OF SENSORY INFORMATION
AND MEMORY STORAGE

Presumably the neural pathways composing these cortical areas involved in the processing of new sensory information undergo rapid modification to accommodate a constant flow of incoming data. This would be necessary for new information to be readily absorbed by the brain and sensed in consciousness. According to this hypothesis, information from these sensory structures would immediately be transmitted to memory storage areas where clusters of neurons corresponding to the encoded form of the original sensory input would be simultaneously activated. In accordance with Hebb's ideas, this process would generate a specific pattern of associated cells, duplicating that registered in the sensory cortices. Neurotransmission would be facilitated within this electrical grouping of cells, thus defining a primitive form of the new memory. The neural patterns generated in these deeper brain regions would be more durable than the cortical templates from which they arose. Patterns created within the sensory cortices would be transient and quickly decay. This would be necessary to allow a continuous stream of data to enter the brain and be processed rapidly. The sensory perception areas would not function as lasting sites for memory storage. They would only provide a temporary repository for data, allowing these to be briefly displayed in consciousness. A more permanent record of the new information would be created by its transfer into the memory storage regions of the brain. A memory generated in this way could only regain entry into consciousness at a later time by passage back into one or more of the sensory cortices. This would occur during memory recall.

Newly imprinted memory traces created during this process might experience several fates. Repeated stimulation of the primitive structure would strengthen the neural circuit, making the engram more durable. In effect, continual usage of such an entity would promote consolidation. Those not frequently activated would be gradually lost from memory. This might occur through spontaneous decay or might involve an active process, as will be discussed later. In this way, the more important, frequently repeated events in our lives would be reinforced in memory, while the mental record of trivial things would gradually disappear. In subsequent chapters, these ideas will be expanded and justified as completely as possible.

MEMORIES AS "STACKED" STRUCTURES

It is proposed here that the structures that compose memories may exist in *stacked* fashion. In effect, similar engrams might overlap each other,

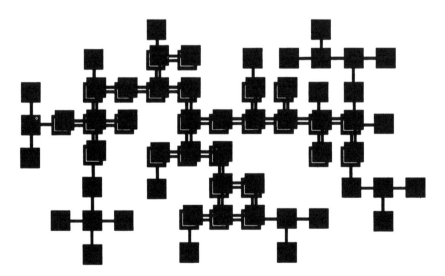

Figure 1.2 In this figure, the concept of "stacked" memories is illustrated. Each square represents a neuron connected to other neurons in the same memory by synaptic linkages. Note that the two memories shown here (designated by black and gray squares) "overlap" each other (i.e., their "paths of neurotransmission" coincide in areas of similarity). In the intact brain, it is postulated that many such memories may overlap, and the structure may be many layers deep.

sharing common neurons in areas of similar electrical or physical structure. In a scheme like this, any given neuron or cluster of neurons might be a functional part of numerous individual memories. The ideas presented earlier suggest that each engram would be defined by a specific path of neurotransmission linking the involved neurons. In essence, a single neuron might be common to many specific paths of neurotransmission and, as such, be shared by numerous memories. A cluster of neurons might have within it many interwoven paths of ionic conduction, each utilizing many common cells and representing a specific memory. A relatively small number of neurons might be capable of encoding a great many memories considering the multiple ways their synaptic connections could be arranged. The idea that memories are structurally or electrically overlapped in common regions also provides a theoretical basis for the conversion of specific memories to generalized form. This is of critical importance to the hypothesis presented here and will be discussed in the next chapter. The concept of *stacked memories* is illustrated in Figure 1.2.

ASSOCIATED UNITS OF MEMORY

It is common knowledge that memories seem to trigger more memories. One thing may remind us of another, and so forth. Memories produced in this way do not seem to be random but probably represent the things that are associated together in nature. This suggests that there may be physical linkages between the structures that code for the events we see as related in experience. Mental organization would thus be based upon neural patterns created and maintained by association linkages. These connections would bond neurons together, creating discrete memories that again might become linked in groups to define even larger units of associated knowledge. Synaptic linkages arranged in this way should be capable of reflecting the many complex relationships encountered in life.

There seems to be ample evidence that events that occur together in experience become associated as memories. A good example of this involves the death of President John F. Kennedy. Virtually all persons who can recall this tragic event can remember what they were doing at the time they heard the news. In most people these memories are strongly linked as a unit and represent an obvious example of association formation between simultaneously occurring events. This type of memory storage is by no means restricted to the major events we witness. Virtually any memory that can be recalled will trigger one or more additional memories, suggesting the extensive association of these entities within the brain. In fact, long chains of memories can be produced by linking one association with the next in sequential fashion. One thing leads to the next, and so on, reproducing the original relationships observed between these items in experience. Once again, this seems to be a direct reflection of the associated organization of memory storage.

It is postulated that our world is recorded in complex patterns of interwoven memories held together by association linkages. This system would allow the relationships we perceive in nature to be maintained in memory. If the events of life were stored as random memories, their natural relationships to each other would be ignored. Association provides a way of organizing mental information so that individual memories maintain their original frame of reference. This would allow remembered events to be interpreted in their proper contextual environment. Were memories stored without this associated organization, they might

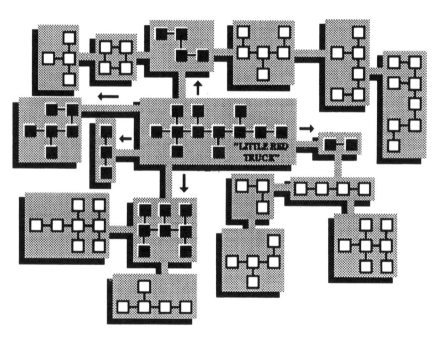

Figure 1.3 In this figure, small squares represent associated neurons that are grouped together in gray rectangles to symbolize memories. Association between these entities is shown by thick gray lines. The visual memory of the "little red truck" has been activated, and its immediate associations have received neurotransmission, as indicated by structures with black-filled squares. Activation of the "little red truck" memory, in the absence of associated memories, would produce only its image in consciousness, without any additional understanding. When its immediate associations are also stimulated, the image acquires a contextual reference, which gives it meaning. Associated memories allow the image of the truck to be interpreted and understood in familiar terms.

have little specific meaning. For example, the isolated memory of a little red pickup truck could mean almost anything. By linking this memory with a specific contextual environment, its relationships to time, place, and specific circumstances would be specified. Such associated memories would serve to define the red truck's relative position within the many entities in memory storage. In other words, the associations of a memory provide it with meaning and therefore serve as its interpretation. This is illustrated in Figure 1.3.

MEMORIZATION AS AN ASSOCIATIVE PHENOMENON

The work presented here is based upon the premise that memory storage involves the formation of association linkages between structures. Various observations about the way we learn seem to support this idea. For example, memorizing a list of unrelated items is often difficult and may require much mental repetition. In contrast, items that are in some way related to each other are often much easier to retain. There are a number of tricks available that often can make a list of unrelated items easier to remember. One technique is to pair the items on the list with memories of things that are already known in a particular sequence. For example, the various landmarks on a familiar street might be mentally linked with the items on the list. We might imagine ourselves placing each item next to the memory of a house, or a fence, or under a familiar tree. The unrelated items are thus placed in a familiar context and associated with things in a known sequence. By recalling each known item of the old list, the things on the unrelated list can also be remembered in proper order. Such mental pairings usually enhance learning and recall.

In associative learning, *preexisting synaptic linkages* may become modified, producing an increase in electrical connectedness between memory components. In this way, the flow of neurotransmission may be facilitated between associated items. In the previous example, conscious visualization of the first list may enable newly associated memories to receive activation energy. The old list may thus serve as a contextual reference, allowing the new list to become electrically integrated into memory. It is presumed here that the items on the random list were *already present* in general memory storage but not previously associated with the landmarks on the street. In other words, things on the second list were already represented in memory in generalized form. Learning simply involved opening the appropriate synaptic linkages joining these preexisting structures. The creation of completely new engrams to represent items on the second list was therefore not necessary. The existence of memories in generalized form is an important concept that will be discussed in the next chapter. In this example, learning probably occurred through a rapid modification of existing linkages between generalized mental elements, thereby enhancing their degree of association. In this way, a coherent memory may have been established.

It is possible that association formation may be a requirement for any event to enter memory storage. Those things that we easily memorize may rapidly make associations with existing memories. This may explain why new events that are similar to things we have experienced in the past are usually easier to understand and remember than completely new, unfamiliar situations. These ideas suggest that the more closely a new event matches past experience, the more easily it will form association linkages and be stored in memory. A mechanism for memory storage based on the formation of association linkages is proposed in the next chapter.

It has been suggested that association linkages bind related memories together within the brain, thus maintaining the relationships derived through experience. It can also be postulated that the strength of such linkages would directly reflect their usage. For example, it would be expected that things frequently encountered together in experience should become strongly associated as memories. In essence, the synaptic connections linking them might become individually more conductive or perhaps would increase in number in response to frequent simultaneous activation. Memories of things less commonly found together should be correspondingly less well associated electrically. This would seem to be a direct consequence of the phenomenon suggested by Hebb and seems to be a way of mentally maintaining the degree to which things are naturally related. Each memory may be linked to numerous other memories with association linkages of varying strengths or numbers as determined by their simultaneous usage in experience. This differential strength of binding should influence the flow of neurotransmission and the activation of subsequent memories. This may actually influence the direction and content of thought.

MEMORY STRENGTH

As postulated, the strength of association between items stored in memory should be a function of their frequency of simultaneous occurrence in experience. The more often they occur together, the stronger their association should become. In addition, the frequent mental recall of the related memories should also increase their strength of association. Repetition seems to be the factor common to both processes. In contrast, memories stored during intense emotion do not seem to require experiential repetition. A single traumatic or very pleasurable event may produce a very durable memory. Perhaps emotion may also produce changes in synaptic linkages but through a different process. This may be a function of the hippocampus and will be discussed in a later chapter.

LIFE EXPERIENCE AND STRENGTH OF ASSOCIATION

Through experience, most memories probably acquire a whole host of associated memories linked with varying strengths. As postulated, this may be a way of ensuring that important or frequently used memories will be stronger and more easily recalled. It seems likely that an activated memory would initially conduct neurotransmission to its most closely connected associations. Perhaps all memories in association with a given entity receive some neurotransmission, but the more tightly bound would receive the most. In this way, those memories of immediate importance should be activated first. Continued activation of the original memory should eventually result in the firing of other associated memories that are less strongly bonded. In this way, most memories' associations could be triggered in a sequence roughly reflecting the strength of their electrical connection to the original memory. The strength of association may thus be a measure of the closeness of relationships encountered in life.

The differential strength of memory association can be directly observed in many ways. If asked to list the important details of a recent luncheon meeting, many facts might be rapidly recalled. It seems likely that those things that most symbolize the meeting will be remembered first, followed by the more peripheral details. Perhaps the food was unusually good, or the speaker's boring presentation was so unremarkable as to be notable. The most memorable thing about the meeting may have been different for each person who attended. It seems probable that the more highly associated memories would be more easily recalled because their synaptic linkages would be more open to neurotransmission.

CHANGES IN ASSOCIATIVE STRENGTH OVER TIME

Over time, a strongly associated memory that falls into disuse may weaken. This is probably synonymous with the process of forgetting. It may be replaced by more current memories with stronger bonding. The flow of neurotransmission would thus be redirected to reflect a new emphasis. In this way, the brain may maintain currency. Memories linked in varying degrees of association may provide us with a filing system that accurately reflects relevant experience. It also provides us with rapid access to stored material, as will be described later.

CHAPTER OVERVIEW

The ideas presented in this chapter form a basis for the hypothesis presented in the remainder of this work. Memories are viewed as clusters of neurons, interconnected by numerous threadlike synaptic projections, which function as ionic channels, creating a pattern specific for each memory. These structures are, in turn, connected to other related memories by more synaptic linkages. Strongly associated memories are linked by more of these fibers or perhaps have synaptic channels that are more electrically conductive. It is proposed that similar memories electrically overlap each other in common areas. As a consequence of this, memories are defined by the path of neurotransmission linking the involved neurons. Any given neuron or cluster of cells may be a functional participant in several pathways of neurotransmission and, as such, may be part of numerous memories. Memory storage seems to involve the formation of association linkages that hold memories in place and designate their relative importance or degree of usage. Because of this associated organization, an activated memory will trigger other memories to which it is closely related. The strength of association bonds may determine the flow of neurotransmission, thereby influencing the direction and content of thought. These ideas will be built upon in subsequent chapters.

Generalization of Memories

Memories have long been recognized as essential to the expression of normal cognitive activity. Despite this, little is actually known of their basic composition or organization within the brain. Some consideration of this subject would therefore seem essential to any reasonable hypothesis of mental function. In this chapter, it is proposed that memories exist as associated units of information from which all mental activity flows.

SPECIFIC AND GENERALIZED FORMS OF MEMORY

Observation suggests that memories can exist in either *specific* or *general* forms. Those that are specific contain information relating to a given time and place. Each is the mental record of a single prior occurrence that has a definable origin in experience. In contrast, general memories have no such specific reference. They seem to represent a conceptualized view of our world acquired over time. A mechanism is proposed in this chapter by which specific memories may progress over time into generalized form. In addition, the relationship of these two general categories of memory to those generally known as *implicit* and *explicit* will be explored.

Generalized memories are common in routine thought and are probably essential to normal mental function. Almost any item encountered in life can be expressed in this form. Such memories seem to be conceptualized representations of similar items or events acquired through prior experience. For example, the generalized image of a house or a tree may be typical of many such items encountered in the past. Complex memories, such as social or professional relationships, can also exist in generalized form. Virtually anything that can be named or described can be expressed in this way. A vast warehouse of such stereotypic composites seems to be present in memory storage and available for use when needed. In this section, a possible origin and physical basis for these generalized memories will be presented.

It is proposed that any situation or event that repeats itself in experience will become generalized in memory over time. This process may occur when many specific memories, which are similar in physical or electrical structure, combine. The resulting memory represents the generalized or *average* of the many specific memories used to create it. In essence, generalized memories appear to represent a blending of many individual memories acquired over time.

GENERALIZED MEMORY COMPLEXES

Throughout our lives, we constantly store new memories that reflect our activities and observations. Gradually these seem to be converted to generalized form, resulting in what might be termed *generalized memory complexes* (GMCs). A great many of these basic units of general information may exist within each of us and are probably critical to normal mental function. The information stored in each complex seems to represent the most common components of all the specific memories used to create it. As such, GMCs provide the brain with a broader type of knowledge than possible with specific memories. The individual events of our lives generate memories containing narrow and well-defined bits of information. In contrast, GMCs contain the extracted and condensed wisdom of experience.

ADVANTAGES OF GENERALIZED MEMORY

Memories stored in generalized form seem to have obvious advantages for the brain. They provide a quick, comprehensive reference for comparison with any situation that might arise. Generalized knowledge not only allows us to accurately predict the outcome of many situations, but also tells us how similar situations have commonly varied in the past. Obviously, this type of information would not be as complete or reliable if only specific memories were available for reference. GMCs can be thought of as summarized versions of past experience, containing only that information that repeats itself on a regular basis. Details that vary frequently from one similar situation to the next are eventually lost from GMCs, leaving only information that is stable and predictable. Any decision based upon this type of knowledge would seem to be much more reliable than that grounded on a single prior experience. Through the use of generalized knowledge, we are able to solve problems, make reasonable judgments, and evaluate life in a predictable way, based on numerous prior similar situations. Without some way of summarizing our experiences, the sheer volume of data in memory storage would be overwhelming. Cognitive analysis would certainly be a slow and arduous process.

GENERALIZED MEMORIES EXIST IN "STACKED" FASHION

The creation of generalized knowledge probably occurs through the storage of memories in *stacked* fashion, as discussed before. All memo-

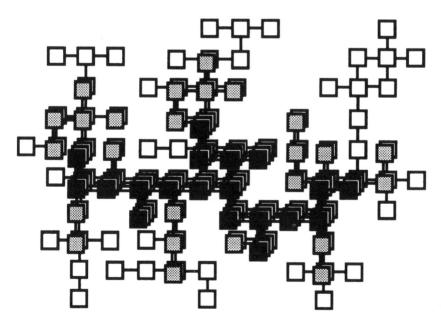

Figure 2.1 "Generalized memory complex" showing differential areas of memory reinforcement. Solid black squares represent associations with the highest degree of reinforcement established through usage. Gray-filled squares represent associations with lesser degrees of usage, and white-filled squares show memory areas with the lowest degrees of reinforcement. For the sake of clarity, only three levels of memory strength have been shown, although many may actually exist. It should be noted that each association (represented here as squares) may contain many individual neurons, which collectively define it as a unit of memory. The strength of synaptic linkages (ability to conduct neurotransmission) corresponds to the degree of reinforcement of involved associations.

ries that share common electrical regions should be capable of undergoing generalization. Each new memory added to an existing complex (GMC) should reinforce any common regions of overlap. Presumably, neurotransmission would become stronger in the synaptic connections linking these shared areas of memory structure. Alternately, new growth of synaptic connections might be stimulated, which may also increase nerve conduction in these overlapped areas. Any noncommon regions of a new overlapping memory would also be stored, but would utilize neurons not shared by the complex as a whole. A stacked GMC is illustrated in Figure 2.1.

FROM SPECIFIC TO GENERALIZED FORMS OF MEMORY

It is a common observation that newly stored memories are usually very easy to recall for a short period of time. For example, the specific details of a typical lunch may remain fresh in memory for a number of hours afterward, but completely fade over the next few days. At the time such memories are stored, it is postulated that strong synaptic connections are created, linking neurons into coherent units specifying the fresh memory. As a consequence, activation and recall should be easily accomplished. At the time of storage, there would be no direct evidence that such a memory had overlapped one or more similar GMCs. Over time, the noncommon regions of this memory should gradually fade or weaken if not reinforced by usage. In contrast, some regions of the stacked memory would become stronger as the GMC was used and new memories sharing common areas were added. Eventually, the less well-reinforced regions of a new memory in such a cluster would disappear, and the fresh entity would blend with the complex. In effect, those specific, nonrepeating characteristics of the memory designating it as a unique individual entity would gradually fade. Its common regions would become part of generalized knowledge, and the new memory would no longer exist as such. In the example used here, a GMC may develop over time specifying the type of food generally consumed at lunch, as well as the general surroundings and circumstances involved. All commonly repeating details of such a typical lunch would become reinforced in memory and become part of generalized knowledge. Individual circumstances for any given lunch may be forgotten, but a generalized representation of a typical lunch will remain in memory. In this way, new memories may progress from specific to general.

Of course the process described is probably not an all or nothing phenomenon. Every GMC would have areas in various stages of deterioration and other regions increasing in overall strength. Both processes would occur simultaneously as GMCs moved toward maturity. These areas of relative strength and weakness would be a direct reflection of the use received by GMCs. In other words, these units of memory would collectively mirror the overall status of the organism at any given time. If conditions changed, altering the content of memories stored, the involved GMCs would be correspondingly modified. In this way our storehouse of generalized knowledge would be constantly updated to reflect the world in which we live.

As suggested, a GMC may arise in response to a recurring similar situation in experience. Each specific memory added to such a complex might be slightly different in some way. Such areas of variability would initially be stored in the GMC, but their long-term survival would depend upon usage. If the variation occurred with some frequency (i.e., if a reasonable number of specific memories added to the complex contained this variation), it would remain a viable part of the GMC. Based upon this reasoning, a generalized memory should retain many of the common variations seen in the situations that become stored in memory. Less frequently occurring variations would be linked to the main body of the GMC with relatively weaker association linkages. In contrast, frequently encountered variations would be strongly linked. Variations with very little or no recurrence would eventually fade completely. In this way, a GMC would contain information about a wide range of similar situations that contained some degree of variation. In addition, the relative linkage strength of different areas of the GMC may provide the brain with some estimate of the probability of occurrence of any given variation. The utility of such information seems obvious. The wealth of knowledge stored in an average GMC would thus be vastly superior to a given specific memory. It seems likely that generalized knowledge greatly facilitates the interpretation of the events in our lives. The conversion of memory from specific to general is illustrated in Figure 2.2.

Although many specific memories never seem to completely fade, the majority of information we process probably undergoes this transition to generalized form. There seems to be an ongoing process of remembering and forgetting as parts of GMCs grow while others deteriorate. At any point in time, our storage of generalized knowledge reflects the overall environment. Changes in our lives are mirrored by corresponding modifications in our storage of this type of knowledge. In effect, there is a dynamic equilibrium at work that continually strives to update our view of the world.

The conversion of specific memory to generalized form seems to be a way of *condensing* large amounts of data. Even so, literally hundreds of

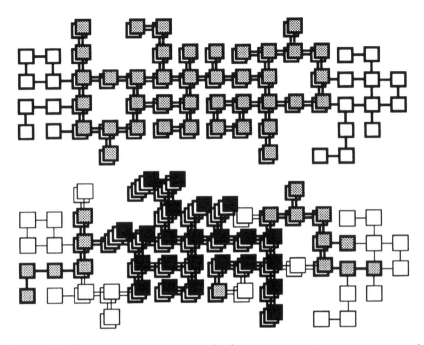

Figure 2.2 In the top structure, two memories (squares represent one or more neurons) overlap in the early stages of generalized memory complex formation. Over time, the components of this structure, which are not reinforced through subsequent experience, fade and weaken, while other parts of the structure become reinforced through usage or the addition of overlapping memories (bottom figure). GMC formation is postulated to be a continuous process of addition and subtraction of component elements.

thousands of GMCs must exist in each of us. In our daily lives, we encounter countless small situations that are recognized and interpreted by the use of GMCs. In a sense, generalized knowledge is a way of cataloging and condensing information so that it can be quickly accessed for reference in such situations. One of the keys to this process appears to be repetition. Any experience that repeats itself should enter generalized knowledge. Its durability as a memory would be a direct reflection of its frequency of usage. In this way, things that are pertinent and current in our experience occupy a prominent place in our brains.

GENERALIZED KNOWLEDGE REPRESENTS REPEATING PATTERNS

Generalized knowledge allows us to sort through the many experiences of our lives and recognize patterns of events that repeat themselves.

Such patterns are represented in memory by those areas within GMCs that overlap and reinforce each other. It is not uncommon for life events to repeat in one way or another over time. Often situations that are basically similar may initially seem confusing because of minor variations between them. Identifying and understanding the common elements may be difficult on first analysis. Over time, such situations often seem to spontaneously clear as the more important and relevant details emerge from the mass of confusing trivia. In such cases, GMC formation may be occurring, allowing recognition of underlying patterns. Through repetition, the basic elements of similar situations may become reinforced, while those with some degree of variation may dissipate. In this way, a clearer picture may surface, allowing us to recognize the stable and pertinent elements involved.

The recognition of patterns in the events of our lives is essential for virtually everything we do. When doctors examine patients, they are searching for patterns of symptoms and physical findings that correspond with various illnesses. Through experience, they have learned which indications are potentially relevant and which are nonspecific or trivial. A doctor's skill lies in being able to recognize the correct patterns from the many things he or she may observe. In many cases, he or she must sort through a multitude of less relevant details to arrive at the proper diagnosis. In contrast, most medical students can name symptoms for a wide range of illnesses but often lack the experience to determine which are clinically relevant. Through repetition, these skills are developed. A wide range of GMCs emerge through training that provides the student with the tools necessary to practice medicine. The specific memories acquired in medical school gradually become generalized as training continues. This progression from specific to general knowledge is critical in the development of any skill and is directly related to this conversion of knowledge.

There are multiple examples of the transition of knowledge from specific to general in our lives. Most new concepts are learned initially by the analysis of specific examples. After a number of these have been considered, the general principles that underlie each blend to provide general knowledge, applicable to a wider range of situations. As any chemistry or physics student understands, working many specific textbook problems leads to a more general understanding of the principles involved. The acquisition of any new body of information follows this same process of knowledge consolidation. As this book is read, new ideas are presented that repeat themselves in various ways throughout its pages. This repetition leads to the formation of new GMCs that serve to categorize the information in the readers brain. Through the process of consolidation, information is converted to generalized form. This process allows the main principles presented here and repeated in various ways to become *highlighted* in the reader's brain. It is my hope that a coherent, clear picture will develop as overall understanding progresses to maturity through the process described.

GENERALIZED KNOWLEDGE AND PREDICTIONS

Another important feature of generalized knowledge is its ability to allow us to make predictions. For the common problems we encounter frequently, generalized complexes will exist. Each GMC coding for such a problem will contain all the common variations encountered, as discussed previously. In addition, GMCs containing information about our prior responses to problems should also be present in memory storage. Each previous action repeated with any frequency will be present for reference. Other GMCs will tell us of the success or failure of our chosen actions in response to various situations. In effect, generalized knowledge stores information that can be used as a reference for numerous situations we routinely experience. By employing this knowledge, we can predict the outcomes of many situations we encounter, and can initiate actions that have proven successful in past similar circumstances. Obviously, generalized knowledge is an important factor in helping us select appropriate actions under different circumstances. It is also a basic component in the process of problem solving. But what about situations we encounter that have no direct past reference in experience? Is it possible to properly interpret them and initiate appropriate actions without a direct reference in memory? In situations such as this, GMCs may be combined to yield approximate solutions that may provide some degree of understanding. This will be discussed in a later section.

SCRIPTS AND SCHEMATA

The description of *generalized knowledge* presented here is similar in many ways to what has previously been referred to as *scripts* or *schemata* (Schank, 1982; Schank & Abelson, 1977). These terms refer to a form of overlearned knowledge that represents a composite of memories for events with similar content and, as such, seem to represent *standardized, generalized episodes*. As proposed for generalized knowledge, elements of the script would be a blend of those derived from its individual component memories. Any aspect of an individual component episode that deviated from the main theme of the script would be retained as a distinct entity. In these respects, generalized knowledge and scripts are similar. Unlike scripts, generalized knowledge is characterized as containing *any type of repeating information* that may arise from life events, as well as cognitive reflection. Generalized knowledge is viewed as a global form of mental organization that is essential to all aspects of normal cognitive function. In essence, generalized knowledge is characterized as having a wider and more comprehensive role in mental activity than scripts and schemata.

SIZE OF GENERALIZED MEMORY COMPLEXES

GMCs have been described as grouping of similar, individual memories that evolve over time and eventually come to represent a composite of the most typical situation. Through this evolutionary process, specific memories are transformed into generalized knowledge that has greater utility as a standard by which to measure the current events of our lives. But what determines the size of any given GMC? Is this an arbitrary decision by the brain, or are there factors that govern the ultimate size of such a complex? From the previous discussion, it should be obvious that GMCs can represent small objects such as trees, cars, houses, and so on, or can contain knowledge of more complex situations, such as interpersonal and professional relationships. In effect, GMCs have a wide range of sizes. It seems probable that the ultimate size of a GMC will be determined by its use in our experience. Anything that repeats itself as a unit, be it small or large, should eventually undergo generalization.

Any single object encountered frequently in our environment should eventually form a GMC. Although it may appear in many settings, its general consistency from one place to the next allows it to undergo generalization. In a like manner, a grouping of small, generalized units that frequently occur together may become linked in association to eventually form a larger, generalized memory. For example, we are all familiar with types of furniture usually found in a bedroom, or appliances in the typical kitchen. In these cases, individual small GMCs have become associated through experience to form larger, stable complexes. The composition and size of any GMC will thus be a direct reflection of the natural grouping of objects or events in nature and their repetition as a unit. And so the formation of generalized complexes is not an arbitrary process but is actually a reflection of life as we see it. Through this process, things are categorized and grouped as they occur in experience.

MAXIMUM SIZE OF GENERALIZED MEMORY COMPLEXES

As indicated earlier, the maximum size of a GMC should be determined by the number of entities that group together and repeat themselves in experience. Based upon this, we can assume that there are probably many more small GMCs than large. This follows when we realize that small, simple situations in life are more likely to repeat themselves than complex affairs with multiple events. In fact, it is probably safe to assume that as GMCs get larger, they become less frequent in number. Eventually they probably reach a maximum size. At this point, life events become too complex to repeat themselves with any significant frequency. Beyond this, large, complex situations are stored as fresh memories that never totally undergo generalization as intact units and may eventually fade. In this way, maximum GMC size is also dictated by naturally occurring circumstances.

MINIMUM SIZE OF GENERALIZED MEMORY COMPLEXES

It seems likely that the minimum size of GMCs is also determined through usage. Many objects or simple events in our lives repeat themselves in virtually the same way each time they are encountered. Such entities may form stable memory units that are rarely if ever divisible in experience. Although they may be components of numerous larger memories, they still maintain their constancy in each setting in which they appear. In effect, they function as minimum units of memory, which retain their identity even though they may be recombined in numerous ways with many other memories to create large GMCs. Their constancy in experience results in stable GMCs, which are always seen by the brain as single, repeating units. They are not necessarily small physical objects or simple events. The only criterion for their existence is that they rarely, if ever, appear in simpler form. Most of the routine objects in our environment exist in this way and form this stable, minimum type of repeating memory.

GENERALIZED MEMORY COMPLEXES
AND MENTAL IMAGES

When new mental imagines are created through the process of imagination, many small GMCs and specific memories may become grouped in association. This general process can be illustrated if we envision a room full of furniture. Each item within such an image would be represented in the brain by a GMC derived from many prior examples of furniture. In some cases, the actual memory of a specific item might also be included. The placement of furniture within this mental room will be guided by the way GMCs have become linked through prior experience. For example, a chair might be envisioned as being next to an end table, which might support a lamp, and so forth. These are common arrangements that would exist in generalized knowledge because they exist in our environment. The general concept that mental images can be constructed by the recombination of smaller units of information, arising from memory, is known as *generativity* (Corballis, 1989; Kosslyn, 1987) and will be discussed further in Chapter 4.

Mental images may be created through a selective and rapid modulation in the synaptic channels that link small units of visual memory. In other words, the creation of a new image may occur when bits of visual memory become *more highly associated* through changes in local neurotransmitter flow. If the items within such an image are mentally rearranged, a new pattern of association would result. It is therefore proposed that mental pictures generated through imagination consist of generalized and specific memories held in place by specific arrangements of association linkages. By the rapid manipulation of the synaptic channels linking these component pieces of information, different images with corresponding associative patterns will result. Such a process may represent a central mechanism that provides the mental flexibility necessary for thought and other cognitive processes.

GENERATION OF FANTASIES

Association linkages are an integral part of memory structure. They allow random neurons to be linked in meaningful ways to create memories. Small GMCs, or fresh memories stored in overlapped fashion, can recombine to create even more extensive entities. In this way, the information in large sensory perceptions can be accurately encoded to preserve the relationships present. Fantasies, which arise from imagination, seem to be various groupings of memory units arranged in new ways and held together by association linkages. This is exactly analogous to the creation of visual images described in the previous paragraph. The generation of fantasies is a unique process that involves more than the mere recall of memories. In addition to visual images, fantasies often contain a mixture of memories arising from different sensory modalities. Complex scenarios can be created at will, which twist and turn in many directions by the manipulation of small component elements. Apparently, in some way, bits and pieces of memories can be recombined and linked in association to tell new stories.

Fantasies often express our internal desires and frequently represent our expectations of the world. They can be reality-based, as when we plan for the future, or completely fanciful, serving no purpose other than the achievement of some pleasurable emotional state. Their formulation occurs at a conscious level, using bits and pieces of events stored in memory. Within our brains are many brief events and longer scenarios acquired through experience. Some of these are stored as GMCs and others are memories of single, unique situations. It is from this rich storehouse that we derive our inspiration for fantasies. Through a process described in more detail later, individual elements of the fantasy are extracted from memory one at a time and linked in association. The final story is based on what we perceive from prior experience to be desirable and to express our feelings at that time. In effect, we are creating synthetic situations that have not been actually experienced. Such compositions may serve many purposes.

If mentally repeated, fantasies will become reinforced exactly as authentic events and will enter memory storage. A fantasy repeated over time with slight variations could conceivably even enter generalized knowledge. This is probably not an uncommon occurrence. Most of us have long-held dreams and expectations of the future that may have begun as fantasies. Through the years, they may undergo modification, forming the basis for generalized knowledge. This is a cognitive process meditated through consciousness.

LINKING GENERALIZED MEMORY COMPLEXES TO FORM MEMORIES

In the previous paragraphs, the formation of mental images and fantasies was discussed. It was postulated that this process involves the linking of various GMCs through the selective and rapid modification of synaptic connections. In this way, preexisting memories may be organized into coherent patterns perceived as images or multisensory scenarios. If frequently repeated, mental events generated in this way should become stabilized in memory in exactly the same way as any other new memory. Presumably the synaptic changes generated in this process would become more permanent through their repeated activation. These ideas seem reasonable for images and scenarios generated totally from preexisting internal components, but what about the memories of events arising from external sensory perception? Could the conversion of incoming sensory data into memories also involve the manipulation of GMCs, as postulated for those mental entities that arise solely from imagination? These questions will be considered.

As suggested in the last chapter, memory storage may begin with the selective modification of existing association linkages. Perhaps this phenomenon can be better understood by reviewing ideas that have already been presented. When new information enters the sensory perception areas, coherent patterns representing these data may be generated in the cells of each structure. As suggested before, conscious awareness of the perception may arise at some point in this process. Patterns generated in this way would then be transmitted to memory storage for comparison with the generalized knowledge stored there. Regions of the incoming perception would be matched with existing structures that corresponded structurally or electrically. Through this process, the overlapped matching regions would receive sufficient energy to become activated. This probably happens very rapidly, stimulating many GMCs to fire almost simultaneously. Because of the near-synchrony of this activation, the electrical connections between these GMCs would be selectively strengthened, increasing their degree of association. This, of course, is basically consistent with the original ideas of Hebb. In this way, new memories would be created by selectively linking parts of older memories and GMCs. This is illustrated in Figure 2.3.

The proposed process works only because of the generalized nature of the information in memory storage. GMCs have an inherent flexibility that allows them to tolerate some variation in the structures they will overlap. It is therefore not necessary for generalized complexes to match bits of incoming data exactly. This is a major strength of the proposed system and will be discussed in more detail later. Sections of the new data need only make approximate matches to overlap and activate GMCs. The new memory is thus stored in stacked fashion with those GMCs to which it most closely corresponds. These units would become sequentially linked in association with each other because of their near-simultaneous activation. Through this process, sections of the new memory would be joined as they appeared in the original perception. In effect, the patterns generated in the sensory cortices would be copied in memory by linking matching units of existing memory. These ideas may explain, in part, how new memories are encoded utilizing generalized knowledge in combination with association linkages. This may be the basic process that underlies all memory storage in the human brain.

In the process described, the synaptic channels linking GMCs are selectively modified (presumably through changes in the amount of

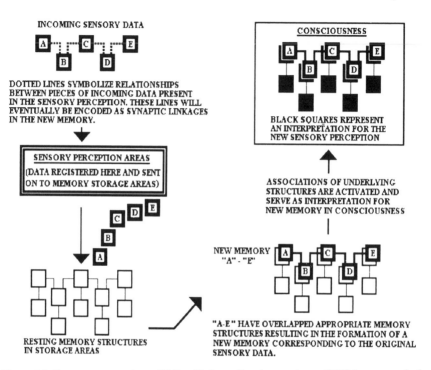

Figure 2.3 Squares represent small bits of information (memories or GMCs) composed of many neurons. Lines connecting these squares represent synaptic linkages. In the upper-left corner of the figure, an incoming perception is shown entering a sensory perception area. These data rapidly flow to memory storage, where matching and overlapping to existing structures occurs. Through this process, unused or underlying synaptic linkages are strengthened, and a new, weak memory of the incoming data is established. It is postulated that each neuron in the brain may have many synaptic linkages that are available to participate in memory formation as illustrated here. As a consequence of this process, the associations of matched structures are activated and serve as an interpretation for the new data. This interpretation is shown in consciousness (upper-right corner of figure).

neurotransmitter released), allowing specific memories to be encoded. In this way, a sensory perception may be converted into a fresh memory. Over time, this new entity may undergo a number of changes. If not re-inforced, the association linkages connecting the various parts of the memory may dissolve, and it will fade. If the memory is reinforced by frequent recall, it may become more durable and survive for a longer time. Alternately, if more similar memories are stored, it may enter generalized knowledge and lose its specific identifying features. At this point, a generalized complex would form. Conceivably the new GMC created in this way might again enter association with other GMCs, forming an even larger complex. It is probably an important concept that generalized knowledge grows by the sequential linking of smaller GMCs that serve as building blocks. In this way, large concepts grow from simpler ideas.

It has been noted by others that associative memory can be conceptualized as consisting of elementary symbols or subunits that can be organized in various ways to create a functional form of neural architecture (Anderson, 1970; Cooper, 1974; Hopfield, 1982; Kohonen, 1977; Palm, 1980; Willshaw, Buneman, & Longuet-Higgins, 1969). Each basic unit in such an arrangement may be represented by one or more electrically connected neurons. It is suggested that such units are similar or identical to the small GMCs that have been conceptualized here.

FLEXIBILITY OF GENERALIZED MEMORY COMPLEXES

The conversion of specific knowledge into generalized has been described in this chapter. In this process, incoming perceptions are electrically overlaid onto matching GMCs to encode specific memories. This is an important step in the overall process, which deserves further comment. The matching process itself seems possible only because GMCs are utilized. By their basic nature they are *very general*. They are a composite of many similar memories from prior experience. Because of this, they do not need to match an incoming perception exactly. Some variation is tolerated, allowing matches to be made that are not exact. In contrast, if incoming perceptions were required to match specific memories, few matches would be possible. Only perceptions identical to a stored memory would match in such a system. An arrangement like this would not have the flexibility to accommodate the almost-endless combination of situations that can arise in life and must be stored in memory. As indicated earlier, the flexibility of GMCs is probably the single most important aspect of generalized knowledge allowing fresh memories to be stored.

THE CONCEPT OF GENERALIZED MEMORY IS NOT NEW

It has long been recognized that memory generalization is probably essential for successful cognitive function. Only through such abstraction can events in memory be freed from specific contextual constraints to provide a general and flexible reference for other related situations. The idea that generalization occurs as a consequence of neural architecture that allows similar memory structures to overlap has been proposed by others. Cooper (1974) and Kohonen (1977) demonstrated that a set of overlapping associative patterns can produce an abstraction that appears representative of the essential features of such a group. Other work, which addresses the generalization of associative memory from different theoretical perspectives, has been published (Ackley, Hinton, & Sejnowski 1985; Fukushima, 1980; Rosenblatt, 1961). A recent discussion of this subject is provided by von der Malsburg (1990).

STIMULUS GENERALIZATION

As indicated, the localization and matching of new data to stored memories appears to be heavily dependent upon an inherent flexibility in the system. Some variation between compared entities seems to be tolerated, and perhaps even necessary, to allow significant matching to occur. The outward manifestations of this phenomenon may have been observed for many years by those who study learning. Pavlov's experiments showed that a dog, conditioned to the tone of a tuning fork, would also respond to the ringing of a bell, the sound of a buzzer, or the click of a metronome. In other words, a second stimulus, which was sufficiently similar to the original conditioned stimulus, would often elicit the conditioned response. The degree to which this occurs has been shown to be in direct proportion to the similarity of the conditioned stimulus to the second stimulus. The phenomenon has been extensively investigated through the years and is known as *stimulus generalization* (Pavlov, 1927).

This phenomenon of stimulus generalization may be a consequence of the flexibility that seems inherent in generalized knowledge. In Pavlov's experiments, similar sounds may have initially been registered in a single GMC because of the nonspecific nature of these entities. Such a generalized unit may thus have been overlapped by any one of several stimuli capable of producing the original conditioned response. In such experiments, discrimination between similar stimuli will eventually occur if additional training is given. Perhaps the various regions of the GMC representing the different stimuli become reinforced through continued repetition. As a consequence, each part of the generalized structure might become more distinctive, enabling similar sounds to be differentiated.

Stimulus generalization is generally explained along the lines of the *identical elements theory* proposed by Edward L. Thorndike early in this century (Thorndike, 1903; Thorndike & Woodworth, 1901). Learning is viewed as a function of *sets of stimulus elements* that can be paired with various responses through training. Activation of a group of stimulus elements would lead to the conditioned response associated with that grouping. The exact nature of each stimulus will be determined by the various elements that compose it. Different sets of stimulus elements might share common features and therefore might contain areas of similarity. If two such groups of elements showed a sufficient number of common features, then a response paired with one stimulus grouping might also be elicited by the other, similar stimulus. Numerous experiments have demonstrated that the higher the percentage of elements shared by the two stimulus groups, the more easily stimulus generalization occurs (Bass & Hull, 1934; Hovland, 1937). This general principle is illustrated in Figure 2.4.

In many ways, these older ideas are compatible with those presented in this work. Stimulus elements may be *identical* to the many small GMCs or memory traces that are postulated here to be linked in association to form progressively larger units of memory. These ideas suggest that an incoming perception would need to overlap a sufficient number of common associations for a stored memory to be completely localized and activated in the matching process. Perceptions with fewer common elements might produce lesser degrees of memory activation. In other words, a perception would be defined by how closely it matched the associations of a memory. Through this process, a current situation might be viewed as only roughly similar to one from the past, or per-

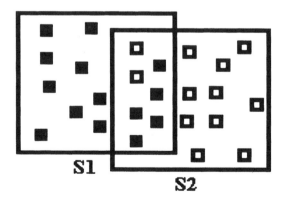

Figure 2.4 S1 and S2 are stimulus populations. Each contains stimulus elements, as indicated by the small squares. As the number of elements shared by the two groups increases (as shown in the overlapped area), S2 will increasingly stimulate the conditioned response paired with S1.

haps almost identical, as determined by the degree of overlap. Analogies might be realized, and subtle similarities between many situations might be recognized through such a mechanism. Obviously this phenomenon may have great utility in the overall process of learning and understanding. Stimulus generalization may therefore be an integral part of the localization and matching process and allow the brain to make direct comparisons between memories or between memories and sensory perceptions. It may also be the basis for the flexibility inherent in generalized memories, as alluded to earlier.

THE ENCODING SPECIFICITY PRINCIPLE

In 1973, Tulving and Thompson suggested the *encoding specificity principle* (ESP) in an attempt to explain *recall* and *recognition* as parts of a single retrieval system. These authors postulated that the retrieval of information depended upon the degree of overlap between elements of the encoded memory representation and those present in the incoming cue. These ideas are, of course, similar to those presented here as well as in earlier work on stimulus generalization. Although this work seemed to answer many theoretical questions about retrieval, it indicated that recall and recognition were *independent* of each other. To explain this lack of relationship, it was concluded that these entities each had differing features that were involved in overlap. In subsequent work, various objections to the conclusion that recall and recognition are independent have been raised (Hintzman, 1992; Santa & Lamwers, 1974). Any relationship that may exist between these two parameters seems to be still in question.

STIMULUS DISCRIMINATION

Of course, if stimulus generalization were permitted between memories with only minimal similarity (i.e., between memories with only a few matching GMCs), many misperceptions and errors in judgment would occur. A boy might become alarmed at the sight of his mother's white fur stole because of its similarity to a white rat, which he had learned to fear. In this case, stimulus generalization would produce an apparent misperception. According to learning theory, *stimulus discrimination* is the process by which similar things become differentiated from each other, and might be viewed as a way of balancing the effects of stimulus generalization. This would be the ability to recognize that two situations were similar but not the same. Obviously, a fine balance between stimulus generalization and discrimination must be maintained to properly appreciate and understand the large amount of data we process daily.

VISUALIZING MEMORIES

If memories could be visualized, they might appear as extensively overlapped patterns of neurotransmission within a matrix of neurons. Numerous GMCs of various sizes would be represented by areas of increased electrical density. These would be extensively connected by ionic channels reflecting their relationships to each other. Single, fresh memories, not yet existing as generalized knowledge, would be linked to GMCs in overlapping fashion. In places, large complexes might overlap each other, designating common areas. Throughout this maze, numerous association linkages would be in various stages of deterioration or growth, reflecting their use in experience. Some might disappear completely, causing the memory or GMC involved to appear more diffuse. Larger GMCs alone or in combination might be noted to extend through several centimeters of brain tissue. They might consist of thousands of smaller component GMCs linked extensively in association. Memory stored in this way would truly be decentralized. A single memory's component parts might be widely separated but maintain electrical connectedness through association linkages. This scenario is consistent with direct experimentation that suggesting that individual memories have no centralized or discrete locus within the brain.

OVERLAPPING OF GENERALIZED MEMORY COMPLEXES

As indicated, GMCs do not exist in isolation from each other. There may be areas of extensive overlap joining two or more in regions coding for common events. GMCs are essentially large memories and would therefore be expected to align themselves in stacked fashion when common areas were present. It should also be possible for large GMCs to be only partially overlapped. For example, a complex situation that repeats itself may result in a large stacked GMC. If each occurrence of this situation has a slightly different outcome, the memory of each of these differing parts may not overlap. The main body of the GMC would therefore be connected to a number of nonoverlapping regions representing dissimilar areas of the memory. In essence, the original GMC may branch at several points, reflecting frequent variations on the central theme. Obvi-

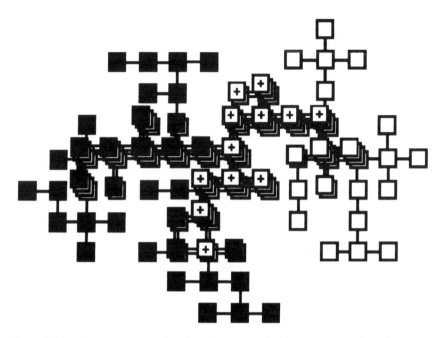

Figure 2.5 In this figure, the overlapping of two generalized memory complexes is shown. One complex is represented by black squares, whereas the other is composed of empty white squares. The cross-marks on some squares indicate the areas where the two complexes overlap each other. The black and white squares represent associations that may each be composed of one or more neurons.

ously the situation can become very complicated. Each GMC may partially overlap many others at various points, and each may have multiple branch points representing small variations in the main scenario. This arrangement would be necessary to reflect the extreme complexity of experience. Once again, this ability of a GMC to contain many variations on a common theme is the basis for much of its flexibility. This is illustrated in Figure 2.5.

MEMORY IN A CONSTANT STATE OF FLUX

A memory storage system utilizing generalized knowledge would be in a constant state of flux. GMCs exist only because of the repetition of similar events. The frequency of this repetition would determine the strength and durability of each complex. There would be a *continual remodeling* process within memory storage areas, reflecting the constant minor and major changes occurring in our lives. Memory storage would mirror these changes through alterations in GMCs and individual memories. A constant process of simultaneous building and deterioration would exist, as described before. Our memories at any given time would reflect our current and recent life experiences.

MEMORIES FROM TWO OR MORE SENSORY MODALITIES

Memories are probably encoded as neural patterns, which are created by specific alterations in synaptic linkages. The paths of neurotransmission established by these activated ionic channels would hold the specific information necessary for the recall of the memory. In a sense, neurons may function only to support and maintain this pattern of electrical connectivity. As proposed earlier, sensory perceptions entering the brain may initially be translated into these types of electrical patterns prior to storage in memory. This may occur in the cortical perception area specific for each sensory modality. For example, an image falling on the retina would be transmitted to the posterior brain and reproduced in the visual cortex. At this point, it still would represent a true image of the original external perception. This information would then be transmitted electrically to memory storage, where the pattern of neurotransmission held in the visual cortex would be reproduced. The association linkages holding this new structure together would be somewhat more durable than those of the cortex, which would rapidly dissolve in preparation for another incoming image. This would seem necessary to maintain a constant flow of data into the brain. Because many perceptions involve two or more sensory modalities, several sensory cortices might be simultaneously active. For example, the image of a rose might be registered separately from its smell and texture, in different sensory regions. Such details would become stored as an individual memory connected by association linkages. Other situational aspects of our encounter with the rose would also be recorded, producing a complex of related memories that might be widely separated from each other. Relationships present in the original perception would thus be reflected and maintained by changes in electrical connectivity joining the various units of generated memory. Through this process, individual sensory perceptions would be electrically grouped in a coherent manner reflecting their simultaneous occurrence in experience. Others have suggested similar ideas. In 1990, Rolls proposed that inputs from different sensory modalities converge at the hippocampus and return to the neocortex via backprojections (feed-

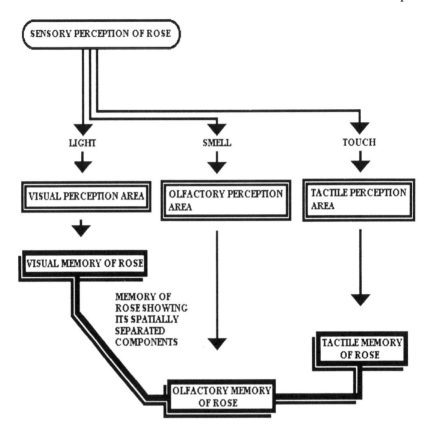

Figure 2.6 It is postulated that the sensory qualities of a rose may be registered and stored in separate regions of the brain, but the overall memory may function as one, coherent unit because of the synaptic projections that join the entire structure. Current research indicates that most memories do not seem to be localized to single, discrete regions of the brain.

back fibers) to produce associated memories. In Figure 2.6, the memory of a rose is illustrated.

MEMORY RECALL AS THE OPPOSITE OF STORAGE

When a memory composed of several separated parts is recalled into consciousness, its circuitry would be simultaneously activated, and the resulting patterns would be electrically transmitted back to the corresponding cortical perception areas. At this point, a reverse of the original translation process would occur. The pattern maintained in memory storage by associative linkages would be generated in the cells of the cortex, and the original perception would be reproduced again for the brain. At this point, a stored memory would become visible in consciousness. For example, the image, smell, and other qualities of a rose would be simultaneously recalled. The reproduction of this memory in various sensory perception areas would generate a conscious awareness of those events that originally stimulated memory formation. The sensory perception areas would not only allow perceptions to be encoded into memories but would also function to reproduce them for the brain when desired. This is dealt with further in the chapter on consciousness.

CLASSIFICATION OF MEMORY

Many schemes for memory classification have been proposed through the years (see Squire, 1987a, for a listing of such systems), which have been based largely on results of testing, as well as natural divisions or dissociations that can be observed in patients with neurological impairment. Because there is generally much overlap between these systems of classification, and because the literature is extensive on this subject, only two of the better-known schemes will be examined in this discussion. Of initial interest here are the forms of memory known as *implicit* and *explicit*. This classification scheme defines memory types on the basis of responses to direct and indirect tests of memory (Schacter, 1987). Explicit tests of memory depend upon the ability to consciously recall previously experienced events. For example, a man may be asked to recall a conversation he had at lunch yesterday, or the circumstances of a previous learning session. Testing is designed to directly test recognition or recall of such knowledge. In contrast, implicit tests do not require the man to recall specific past events. Responses are, instead, based on a store of information that seems to be derived from general experience (i.e., his answers are inferred indirectly from a store of knowledge that is not situationally specific). Whenever an event with a definable origin in time and place is recalled, conditions for explicit memory exist. When facts are recalled that have no association with a identifiable prior experience, implicit memory is utilized. It will be argued here that both implicit and explicit forms of memory may arise from generalized memory complexes.

It has been proposed that GMCs are formed when the neural structures representing similar perceptions "overlap" in electrically compati-

ble regions. Over time, some areas of the structure should become reinforced, while others may weaken, as explained previously. Through this
dynamic state of flux, individual structures should arise that are representative of experiences that are similar and related. Such information
would be general in nature, in that the structures derived in this way
should be the "average" of many similar events. Recall of the information contained by such a neural formation should therefore yield general
information, without reference to single events from experience. In this
regard, such data should be identical to those that have been classified
as *implicit*.

In addition to the *general memory* contained within a GMC, it has
been postulated that new perceptions are also stored at some structural
level. As explained before, such information should remain viable, in
separate and individual form, for some time before being absorbed or
converted to generalized knowledge. Such stored data therefore seems
to meet the criteria for *explicit memory* in that they can provide a reference to specific, identifiable events from the past. It is therefore proposed that the different neural structures corresponding to both implicit
and explicit memory forms are contained within GMCs. Others have
speculated that these two divisions of memory arise from structures of
different neural composition (Graf & Schacter, 1985: Moscovitch, 1984:
Richardson-Klavehn & Bjork, 1988). This idea is compatible with the different structural stages that may be present within GMCs as information
progresses from specific to general.

In 1982, Tulving, Schachter, and Stark demonstrated that implicit
and explicit memory change differently over time when measures of
recognition and priming are evaluated. Retention for explicit memory
was found to be substantially less than for implicit memory, which
showed little decay over time. Such findings are consistent with the
concept of generalized memory presented here, which predicts that explicit memory (new memory or memory that has not yet become generalized) should gradually progress to implicit memory (generalized
knowledge). The relative stability of implicit memory may, of course,
be related to its high degree of reinforcement, as discussed previously.
Such research data suggest a compatibility between the implicit–
explicit memory system and the concept of generalized memory proposed here.

In a second classification system, memory is defined as declarative
(semantic and episodic) or nondeclarative (procedural). This scheme,
which was originally suggested by Tulving (1972, 1983, 1985, 1987, 1989),
attempts to directly characterize the nature of the different forms of
memory in long-term storage rather than classifying it on the basis of

testing. In many ways, this system is similar to the implicit–explicit scheme described earlier. For example, declarative memory is usually considered to be explicit in nature, whereas procedural, or nondeclarative memory, is felt to be implicit. In Chapter 7, this system is discussed in detail in relationship to the memory loss experienced in amnesia.

LANGUAGE AS A SHORTHAND FORM OF SELF-EXPRESSION

The origin of language and it evolution in man are complex subjects for which there is considerable literature. Because of this, no attempt will be made here to review this subject in its full scope. In the following paragraphs, only those ideas with a direct relevance to the association hypothesis will be discussed.

Language seems to be a way of expressing human thought in a concise, symbolic manner. It may have evolved when man developed the ability to manipulate verbal sound in a precise manner. As a result of this new skill, communication became much easier and more rapid. The dissemination of information between people must have increased exponentially in a relatively short period of time. Man's dominance as a species may be a direct consequence of this evolutionary development. Despite this, language may be no more than a shorthand form of self-expression. Rather than evolving as a totally new way of thinking and information processing, it probably arose as an extension of existing, preverbal, cognitive function. Over time, various sounds came to symbolize the common events and objects in life. Language slowly became the communication of choice with others and became interwoven into conscious thought.

Despite its extensive usage today, language might still be considered to be only a symbolic way of expressing inner reality. As such, it would seem necessary for the brain to translate the words it hears into their original meanings for understanding to occur. The reverse of this process would be necessary to express our ideas in words. In this work, language is viewed as a way of expressing our inner, nonverbal thoughts to others. In essence, it converts thought into a form suitable for communication. It is not seen as a replacement for the original form of preverbal thinking but as a supplement that allows its external expression.

The ideas expressed here seem to be a natural extension of the proposition that *things occurring simultaneously in experience become joined in memory.* Words are considered to be verbal sounds that have become paired through frequent usage with defining memories. Language is, in turn, an association of words that facilitates the transfer of complex information. In essence, language is viewed as a shorthand form of communication that developed because of the natural tendency for things to associate in memory. These ideas will be explored here and in the chapter on consciousness.

LANGUAGE AND GENERALIZED MEMORY COMPLEXES

It is likely that the numerous words we employ in communication exist within the brain as GMCs. Through frequent usage, each word may have developed its own *usage profile*. This would include each word's various connotations in different situations, as well as other words or phrases to which it is normally joined in sentences. Each GMC representing a word

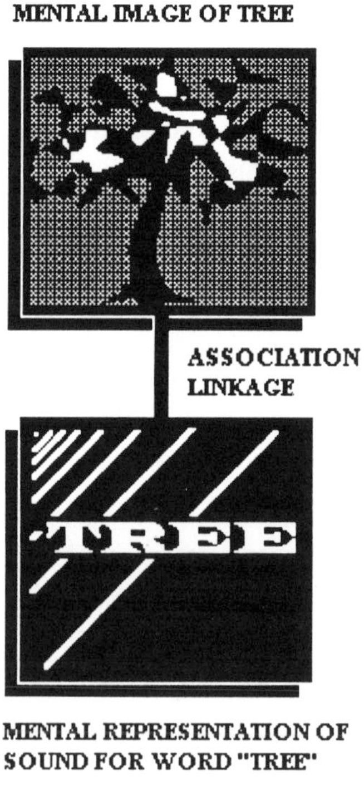

MENTAL IMAGE OF TREE

ASSOCIATION LINKAGE

MENTAL REPRESENTATION OF SOUND FOR WORD "TREE"

Figure 2.7 Through experiential pairing, the memory (GMC) for the image of a tree has become linked with the general memory representation for the sound of the word *tree*. In this way, the sound has acquired a visual association that defines it.

would also be linked in association with memories of sensory data that define its meaning (i.e., the GMC for the sound of the word *tree* would be electrically coupled to the GMC for our stereotypic image of a tree. This is illustrated in Figure 2.7. This type of association would, of course, be a natural consequence of their associative pairing in experience.

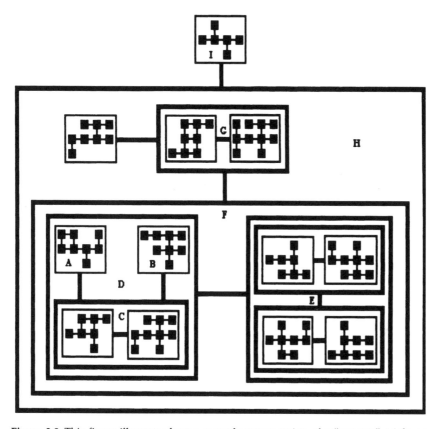

Figure 2.8 This figure illustrates how a mental representation of a "concept" might appear. The smallest squares represent the smallest bits of associative memory. They may be GMCs or nonrepeating, small memories. Each is composed of numerous neurons, which encode the basic memory. Each small square (an association) is linked to another such unit of information, to which it has become linked through experience. Clusters of such associated squares have, in turn, formed stable associations with other such clusters. The process continues until very large and stable units of information become linked in a single complex. Note that each level of association has its own associations, which define the given complex as a whole. For example, A and B serve as defining associations for Complex C but A, B and C, as a unit, serve as an association, which defines Complex E. The large Complex H defines the whole concept. Complex I, in this example, represents the memory of the word that symbolizes the concept defined by Complex H.

CONCEPTS AND GENERALIZED MEMORY COMPLEXES

After many years of evolution, our language contains many words that no longer relate directly to physical reality, but to what might better be termed as mental reality. Words representing such conceptual ideas may be stored as a combination of basic words and smaller concepts. A generalized complex for such a concept probably starts when a few word-GMCs combine, as various aspects of a larger idea become appreciated. Eventually the cluster of interlinked associations would acquire a meaning separate from those of its individual parts. In essence, it would become a large GMC made up of many smaller complexes, functioning as a single unit and having a unique meaning as a group.

It seems reasonable that the meaning of a concept may arise through a collective understanding of the many individual ideas that compose it. In this way, the brain may be able to comprehend abstractions that have only a distant relationship to the physical and tangible information we acquire through the senses. Concepts can therefore be viewed as relatively stable groupings of smaller ideas that have a single, collective meaning as an intact unit. These entities may be structurally represented in memory storage by large GMCs. This is illustrated in Figure 2.8.

WORD AND SENTENCE GENERALIZED
MEMORY COMPLEXES

Language is composed of numerous word-GMCs that can be linked in association in various combinations to form sentences. Over time, certain stable patterns of usage may have emerged. GMCs coding for words that are frequently used together may have become more closely associated. Larger GMCs, representing commonly used groupings of words, would have resulted from this process. In essence, GMCs would exist for words as well as commonly used phrases and even sentences. This would seem to be a natural consequence of the use of language. Each individual might have at his disposal numerous GMCs coding for partial or complete preformed sentences. These would be available to express or interpret the many common ideas that repeat themselves in our experience. The intriguing aspect of this idea is that such a GMC should be capable of tolerating a considerable variation in sentence structure. In essence, a sentence might be phrased in numerous ways and still correspond to a single GMC. This would reflect the general ability of GMCs to store all common variations of a single situation. A sentence arising from a GMC might be verbalized in many different ways because of the inherent flexibility of generalized knowledge.

There is certainly no obvious reason GMCs coding for entire sentences could not exist. Association seems to be a widespread phenomenon that enables things to be mentally grouped as they occur in our lives. This would seem to be as applicable to language as well as to all other events we mentally process. Groupings of commonly used words into association complexes representing commonly used phrases or sentences would enable rapid interpretation as well as expression of language. It seems reasonable that much of our language is stored in this way.

PREVERBAL THINKING

As indicated before, the construction of fantasies may involve the sequential combination of generalized and fresh memories to tell a story. In this way, the recollections of prior events can be reorganized to generate new scenarios not previously experienced. All types of situations can be envisioned. Our unfulfilled hopes and dreams can be mentally realized. We can plan for the future and devise solutions to the many problems that arise on a daily basis. Fantasy can be a brief escape from the stresses of reality but may also serve many practical purposes.

In modern man, verbal thinking is integrated with visual imagery and other sensory data to create fantasies. At a more basic level, language is probably *not necessary* for this process to operate. Although words undoubtedly add a clarifying dimension to our fantasies, they do not appear essential. It is tempting to speculate that thought in preverbal man largely consisted of some version of nonlinguistic fantasy formation. Thinking based solely on the combination of sensory memories is crude by today's standards, but may have been the prime form of thought in early man. Many animals of today probably use some variation of this type of thinking.

The idea that language itself is not necessary for cognitive competence can be illustrated by observing those who have never developed formal language. It is known that illiterate, deaf–mute adults can function in a seemingly successful manner, despite their inability to use language (Lane, 1984). They appear to have a normal ability to accurately remember life events and to store and utilize episodic memory in a framework of conventional consciousness. They can communicate with others through mimicry and understand social relationships and the emotional responses of others. They often hold jobs that require manual skill and the ability to reason. In short, such individuals seem to function in an acceptable and successful manner in the complete absence of a verbal language. Perhaps they use a more basic and ancient *language of thought*, which may have originated in prelinguistic man. This concept will be more fully characterized in subsequent chapters.

SIMILARITIES BETWEEN FANTASIES AND LANGUAGE

There are similarities between the generation of fantasies and the construction language that deserve some comment. Both are ways in which thought can be expressed within the brain (i.e., both are utilized as modes of thinking in modern man). In addition, both seem to arise from the successive linking of GMCs to produce coherent thought. The type of GMC used in each mode is different, but the overall process by which they are joined to create narrative thought appears to be the same. These ideas will be expanded in subsequent paragraphs.

EVOLUTION OF LANGUAGE AS A FORM OF THOUGHT

As postulated, the manipulation of nonverbal mental entities may have been the only way primitive man had to inwardly express his thoughts. Over time, language developed and words began to be used in combination with sensory memories. Rather than displacing the older form of thought, language appears to have supplemented and enriched it. Obviously, both function in combination to produce the concise and expressive form of thinking we now experience in consciousness. The similarities between the generation of fantasies and the construction of language may not be purely coincidental. Language appears merely to be *an extension of preverbal thinking* that arose when our ability to manipulate sound evolved. Both may employ a common mechanism by which association linkages are rapidly modified to produce coherent thought.

Before the development of language, all conscious thought probably involved the recall and recombination of sensory memories. Communication between people probably involved various hand and body gestures in combination with crude, nonspecific sounds. As the human larynx evolved, a wide range of verbal sounds became possible. With continued repetition, certain sounds became paired through association with events and objects from the environment. Through this process, sounds representing words gradually acquired meaning. Conscious thought and communication with others slowly became dependent on language. To utilize this adaptation, it probably would have been necessary to add a *translation step* to the processing of verbal data. In effect, words, which have no intrinsic meaning by themselves, had to be converted into basic terms understandable by the brain each time they were used. Each word had to be translated into its defining associations. Only in this way could these sounds have meaning to the brain. Prior to language, this step was not necessary. Perceptions could be directly compared with memories on equal terms. Understanding was immediate, because memories were encoded in the same terms as used for incoming sensory data. This probably worked well but did not provide for rapid communication with others. Although language probably requires a translation step each time it is used, it greatly facilitates information exchange between people.

In modern man, translation occurs at an unconscious level and consequently is largely out of our awareness. It is a rapid process and occurs each time we hear a spoken word. It follows that a reverse translation process must also occur each time we express our thoughts in words. In effect, we still utilize sensory memories to process information at an unconscious level, but these are converted into a medium applicable to communication with others. Language seems to represent an *interface* between the older brain, which stored and processed everything using sensory memories, and the newer brain, which is capable of direct communication with others. As such, language may not represent a totally new system of thinking, but an addition and refinement to the previous arrangement.

THE DUAL CODING HYPOTHESIS

The idea that neural structures encoding words may be linked with their visual representations in memory was originally expressed by Paivio (1986) in his *dual coding hypothesis*. He postulated that mental activity arose from the interaction of a system specialized to handle visual information (the nonverbal imagery system) and one that dealt only with speech and writing (the verbal system) Within these systems, words were represented by *logogens* and images by structures, which he called *imagens*. He further assumed that these entities were connected by referential links that allowed words to induce both verbal and nonverbal codes. These ideas are similar in many ways to those presented here.

FORGETTING

As indicated in this chapter, the fading of material stored within the variable regions of a GMC is critical to its ongoing maturation. In essence, parts of the memory complex are forgotten, while others are simultaneously strengthened through repetition and survive. Learning theory suggests that there might be several mechanisms by which memories fade or weaken over time. One of the older ideas used to explain forgetting is the *trace decay theory* (Worchel & Shebilske, 1986). According to this hypothesis, memories start out strong, and their strength is maintained through frequent use. Without sufficient repetition, memories gradually lose their structural integrity and become increasingly more difficult to recall. Although this theory is appealing in its simplicity, it does not explain how a seemingly long-lost memory can suddenly be triggered into awareness by some incidental event. Such memories are obviously not lost but seem to have become less accessible to recall over time. Perhaps the access routes to these structures become weakened, rather than the memories themselves.

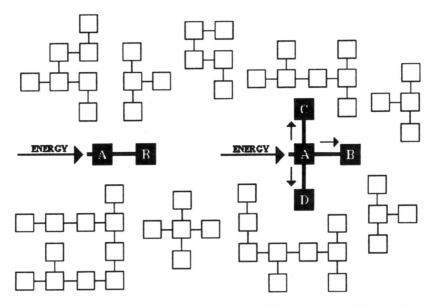

Figure 2.9 This figure illustrates the concept of competitive interference. Energy activating association A in the left part of the figure would be exclusively passed on to B, making it appear to be a strong and easily recalled memory. In contrast, energy arriving at A in the right figure would have three routes it could take and, as a consequence, B would be recalled only one-third as often. B would therefore appear to be weaker or partially forgotten because of this competitive interference. In this example, all synaptic linkages are assumed to be of the same strength.

INTERFERENCE THEORY

An alternate explanation for forgetting comes from *interference theory*, which was first explicitly stated by McGeoch in 1932. McGeoch believed that forgetting did not occur in an absolute sense (i.e., as suggested by the trace decay theory). This idea has now been adopted, at least in part, by many modern neuroscientists. Once an association is established between two items in memory, *A–B*, the strength of this linkage remains intact despite disuse of the association. Any retention loss for this associated pair that occurs over time is the result of new learning that interferes with the original association. For example, if the memory *A* also acquired *C* and *D* as associations, there would be a lowered probability that *B* would be triggered upon the activation of *A*. In other words, the original pairing of *A–B* would be *diluted* by the addition of *A–C* and *A–D*. Neurotransmission originating at *A* would thus have three available paths it could travel, rather than the original single route to *B*. The recall of *B* would therefore be reduced, and it would appear to have been partially forgotten. In actuality, the memory would have experienced a competitive reduction in activation because of the alternative associations. In essence, we could say that the route to *B* had become diluted, even though the association pairing, *A–B*, still existed in memory storage. This is illustrated in Figure 2.9.

PROACTIVE AND RETROACTIVE INTERFERENCE

Through the years, interference theory has been tested extensively with a wide variety of experimental approaches. Two types of interference have been well documented. *Proactive interference* occurs when previously learned data inhibit the acquisition of new material. In contrast, *retroactive interference* is the loss of retention that occurs in older material when new information is stored in memory. In effect, this theory suggests that forgetting, or *memory fading*, may occur when the component parts of a memory become diluted with additional associations as a consequence of new learning. Older data would be competitively weakened by the acquisition of new material and vice versa. Both situations are consistent with the McGeoch's association model. It is conceivable that dilution of this type could result in the total destruction of a memory over time, if it was extensive. As a consequence, forgetting would occur.

FORGETTING AND REMEMBERING
AS ONGOING PROCESSES

Presumably, the strengthening of a memory would involve changes in the basic structure permitting a greater flow of neurotransmission between the component parts. In regions of GMCs undergoing enhancement, *A–B*-type pairings might become strengthened by the addition of more or stronger linkages produced by a repetition of *A–B* in experience. This might be visualized by assuming that the thin linkage between *A–B* would become thicker, or that two or more of these single, thin linkages might be generated as the result of repetition. Either change would be expected to produce an increase in electrical conductivity between the associated entities. In contrast, the increased rate of fading postulated to occur in the variable regions of the GMCs might be due to a reversal of this process, or perhaps to retroactive effects of new learning. If fading were due to interference, the relationships between the numerous *A–B* pairings in the variable regions of GMCs would become diluted by the addition of new associations added to *A* as the result of nonrepeating experience. The net result of memory fading would be a decrease in the electrical conductivity connecting the component parts of the structure. Whatever the mechanisms involved, forgetting and memory enhancement may be simultaneous and ongoing processes reflecting changes in life experience. In effect, similar situations would enhance the strength of a GMCs in certain regions, while the areas of variation within a GMCs produced by slightly different experiences would be weakened. At present, it is impossible to determine the exact mechanism by which these changes occur. Perhaps both are involved to some extent. This idea was expressed by Wickelgren in 1977.

CHAPTER OVERVIEW

In this chapter, the progression of knowledge from *specific* to *generalized form* has been discussed. This seems to be an ongoing process, which provides us with a flexible and easily adaptable type of information for daily use. Generalized knowledge seems to be the basis for language and most of the skills we employ. Without it, we could not interpret the numerous sensory perceptions we encounter almost constantly while awake. It is the basis for memory storage within the brain. It represents a major form of mental organization, which provides the framework for most, if not all, of our mental activities. The units of generalized knowledge have been termed *generalized memory complexes* or GMCs. They can be small or combine to form sizable entities containing large amounts of information. Their size is not arbitrary but is determined by their usage in experience. They are envisioned as clusters of neurons held together by association linkages, which can be strengthened by usage. The basis for all memory formation is the association of various events in our lives with each other. In effect, we store a mental representation of the world as we see it within our brains. This is only possible by linking things in memory that are naturally associated in experience. Things are stored and classified in a way that facilitates their localization and recall. This will be discussed in subsequent chapters. Taken together, these factors provide a reasonable biological basis for the hypothesis presented here.

3

Localization of Memories

Memories constitute a record of past experience. In this capacity, they function as a comparative reference by which current life events can be judged and understood. In effect, memories seem to provide a way of integrating the past with the present so that life might be viewed in proper perspective. It is likely that our memory stores are utilized almost continuously to accomplish this task during waking hours. Obviously an efficient system must be available for the rapid access and retrieval of pertinent data. By organizing memories in associative fashion, such a system seems possible.

When the vast number of memories contained by the human brain is considered, the problem of localization becomes apparent. Retrieving a single memory from the millions in storage would appear to be the literal equivalent of finding the proverbial needle in a haystack. From observation, it seems apparent that the human brain does not locate memories in the same way as do digital analog computers. These machines operate by a process that has been termed *brute force* (i.e., each piece of data is checked in sequence until the desired information is identified). This is obviously time-consuming when the amount of information present is large. In some advanced chess-playing programs, up to one million separate moves may be checked per second by this method until an appropriate selection is made. In contrast, a human chess master may only consider a dozen or so moves that appear relevant at any point in a game. In some way, the number of potential moves has been rapidly narrowed, without the necessity of considering every possibility. Unlike the computer, his memory storage is organized so that every possible move does not need to be considered. He uses a much more sophisticated localization process, which has evolved over millions of years. A possible mechanism for this system is described here. Other theories of memory retrieval have been proposed (Anderson & Bower, 1972; Kintsch, 1970; Tulving and Thomson, 1973; Watkins & Gardiner, 1979).

LOCALIZATION AND MATCHING OF MEMORIES

It is proposed that when a sensory perception enters the brain, a process of *localization and matching* of appropriate similar memories is initiated. This is probably a constant, ongoing process during waking hours to deal with the almost nonstop stream of incoming data we experience. In addition, conscious thought also utilizes this process, as will be described in a later section. The ultimate purpose of this localization procedure is to find relevant memories that serve to identify and interpret incoming information. Each new piece of data can only be understood in light of prior experience, as stored in memory. This internal record of the world serves as a reference by which all new information is judged.

THE FLOW OF NEUROTRANSMISSION DURING MATCHING AND LOCALIZATION

The localization of a memory or GMC by an incoming perception presumably results in its electrical activation. In other words, the merging of the two similar structures during matching may result in the discharge of stored ionic potential to adjacent neurons. It is reasonable to assume that other GMCs and memories in association with the activated structures are the recipients of this energy. As postulated, neurotransmission is probably facilitated between entities that have become associated through usage. And so, it is suggested that when a structure is matched, neurotransmission is conducted to its electrically linked associations. Since each GMC and memory is connected to numerous other structures, this probably results in a widely divergent flow of energy. As will be explained, this is of major importance to the localization of larger structures that are composed of smaller units.

THE MATCHING AND LOCALIZATION PROCESS

The first step in memory localization is probably the comparison of incoming sensory data with structures in memory storage. Patterns created by the activation of neurons in the sensory perception areas by stimuli would be electrically transmitted to memory storage regions. Established memories would then be compared with this new data and activated only if there were significant similarity. Let us consider how this might be accomplished in the visual system. An image falling on the retina would be transported to the posterior brain and reproduced in the visual cortex as a geometrically true representation. The matching of bits and pieces of this visual information to GMCs within memory storage would be rapid (i.e., many individual matches would be made almost simultaneously). As discussed before, individual GMCs and memory fragments localized and activated in this way should associate with each other, producing a primitive new memory corresponding to the incoming data. Some GMCs or memories might be only partially matched or overlapped in this process and thus would not be activated as whole entities. In contrast, structures showing a significant degree of overlap should be completely activated. For example, overlapping would be virtually complete for a familiar image that had previously been stored in memory. Structures identified in this process would, in turn, produce stimulation in their associated memories. Those undergoing subsequent activation would provide interpretation for incoming data. In such a scheme, the flow of neurotransmission coming from the visual cortex would touch many structures in memory storage, but complete activation would occur only in a few. Those memories most closely corresponding to the incoming perception would be the most highly matched and would therefore receive the most stimulation. Associations of those structures that experienced activation would then provide interpretation for the original visual data.

This scenario suggests that memories in storage showing the highest degree of overlap with information coming from the visual cortex would be identified as those most similar to the incoming data. If no specific memory existed for the perception, the structure or structures most closely matching the incoming data might still provide some degree of interpretation. The closer the match between the incoming perception and the available stored material, the more understanding there would be of the new data. In some cases, the match might be so poor as to produce no meaningful interpretation for the perception. This might happen when no stored structure could be significantly overlapped. The matching process would ultimately produce the highest degree of activation in structures with the greatest correspondence to incoming data.

THE STRUCTURE OF MEMORIES

As indicated before, GMCs can be very small or relatively large. A GMC is formed because the associations that compose it vary little in experience. In other words, a GMC remains constant because of repeating experiences that do not differ significantly. As such, GMCs function as discrete units that may have their own set of associations. In effect, a group of small memory structures may form a stable complex which, as a unit, has associations that are specific for it rather than for any of the separate associations of which it is composed. A grouping of such associations may thus have a meaning unique to the stable unit as a whole. This would seem to be an important concept. Consider, for example, 50 small, independent structures such as GMCs or fresh memories. Each of these would have a separate group of associations providing it with an individual meaning. Linked in a cluster representing a larger memory, these small entities may have a combined meaning defined by associations specific only for the group. Such groups may again combine to form even larger units which, once again, would have their own defining associations. Memories, or GMCs, would grow in this way, producing perhaps very large clusters of associated components. At each level, a separate set of associations would provide each structure with its own unique meaning. In essence, small memory units would combine to form larger units, and so on, until memories of maximum size were achieved. This idea was illustrated in Figure 2.8. This would seem to have important implications for the matching process. The smallest pieces of incoming data would initially be matched to the smallest GMCs in memory storage. In this way, memories and GMCs containing these component units would be activated. They would, in turn, combine with other matched units to activate even larger structures. The process would continue until the largest groupings possible could be identified. The associations of these matched units would provide the interpretation for incoming data.

It seems reasonable to assume that events that are associated in experience become physically linked as memories. In this way the relationships observed in nature would be structurally maintained in memory storage. This is a basic tenet of the hypothesis proposed in this work. As mentioned earlier, we can predict that small generalized memories link in association to form larger units, which can again combine to form even larger entities, and so forth. This would seem to be the most natural form of physical organization for a system based upon associations. Memories would therefore be organized in associated units of various sizes, each of which would have its own unique set of defining associations. For any associated unit to fire as a whole, a sufficient number of its component pieces would need to be identified and activated. As small component units become localized and matched to incoming data, larger complexes with sufficient stimulation would become activated. This additive process would continue until the largest units possible corresponding to incoming data were identified. In this way, maximum interpretation of new data would be achieved from stored memories.

STORING NEW MEMORIES

The process described would also function as a way of storing new memories. As identified complexes were activated in *near-synchrony*, association linkages between them should become strengthened. This, of course, is an extension of Hebb's ideas suggesting that the simultaneous activation of memories strengthens their interconnecting linkages. It seems a reasonable assumption that near-simultaneous activation may produce the same results. This idea is further supported by experimental data indicating that near-simultaneous activation of afferent nerve pathways is sufficient to produce long-term potentiation (McNaughton, Douglas, & Goddard, 1978). This phenomenon is thought to be important to some forms of memory storage and will be discussed more fully later in this section. If a pattern of GMCs matched in this way corresponded to that of an existing memory, the shared linkages should become stronger through this process. If the pattern of GMCs matched did not fit an existing structure, a new memory would result by the incorporation of existing but unused linkages connecting the involved entities. The creation of a new memory would thus involve the strengthening of any shared linkages or the recruitment of new linkages where necessary.

The net result of the process described would be a specific ordering of existing, small GMCs to define a new, larger structure. In this way, a new memory would be encoded and its associated component units established. The new entity might completely utilize small component parts already present, or in some cases might be partially stored in neurons with no prior organization. This would occur if some pieces of new data could not be matched from prior experience. Were there no provision for the storage of unique data with no prior reference in memory, the system would be impractical. There would be no way for totally new information to be learned or incorporated into memory. In the proposed system, old memories would be reinforced and new ones established in the same process. According to this model, memory localization and storage would operate simultaneously. New perceptions would thus be identified and stored in memory by the same basic process. This concept was discussed earlier and is illustrated in Figure 2.3.

At this point, let us examine in more detail the suggested mechanism by which new memories are created and stored. As proposed, incoming information would be registered within the sensory perception areas in patterns corresponding to the original input. These data would then be electrically transported to memory storage and matched to the most elemental GMCs and bits of memory present. Many of these entities would already be extensively linked as functional parts of numerous larger memory elements. Each small unit of memory localized in this process would receive stimulating energy and undergo activation. In rapid order, many small memory structures would be identified and activated in this way. The near synchrony of this process would serve to link sequential pieces of the new memory in association. It is proposed that this process increases the conductivity between the involved neurons, as proposed by Hebb over 40 years ago. Through this process, a new memory would be created by the reordering of preexisting small memory units into a pattern specific for the incoming perception. This process would be possible because of rapid modifications in the ion channels linking the involved units of memory. The entity created at this point would be fragile and transient. Further processing would be required to produce a more durable structure. The consolidation of such entities into longer term memories will be considered later.

VISUALIZATION OF NEW MEMORIES

A new memory created in this way might be visualized as a series of small component units held in a specific arrangement by association linkages. The new structure thus formed might overlap many older memories to one degree or another. In some areas, large GMCs or strongly reinforced memories might be partially overlapped, while in other regions weaker structures might be involved. As a consequence of this arrangement, the new memory should have regions in which its connecting linkages would be very strong because of the underlying structures and other areas composed of relatively weak linkages. This would be a natural consequence of a system in which component parts and connecting linkages were shared by several memories. In addition, some regions of the new memory might not overlap existing memories at all but be imprinted on unused neurons. The strength of these regions should be that of the new memory itself, without the influence of pre-existing structures. Without any underlying prior memory structure to provide strength, bonds formed in this way would probably be very weak in most cases. Based upon this mechanism, it might be predicted that the typical new memory would be *stronger* in certain regions and *weaker* in others. This is another way of saying that the electrical connect-

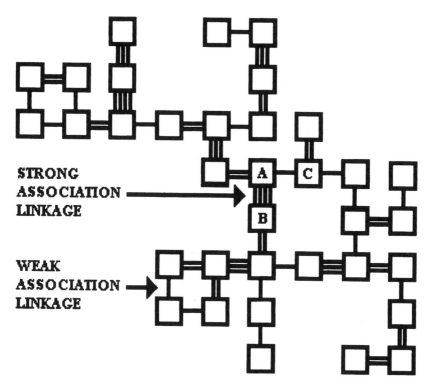

Figure 3.1 In this figure, a memory with differential regions of strength is illustrated. Squares represent neurons that compose the memory. Lines connecting squares represent synaptic linkages. Neurons connected by single lines are less well associated than those with more than one linkage. For example, A and B are connected by several lines, indicating strong association (high electrical conductance), whereas A is only weakly linked to C. High electrical conductance between neurons probably results when multiple memories, which share common connections, are overlapped, or a single memory is frequently reinforced. A new memory may overlap such established structures and should acquire the relative strengths and weaknesses that are present, as explained in the text.

edness of a new memory would not necessarily be homogeneous from one region to the next. The practical significance of this would be that parts of large memories might not show the same degree of retention on recall. In other words, some parts might be more easily remembered than others. A new memory, displaying differential areas of strength as conceptualized here, is illustrated in Figure 3.1. These ideas will be expanded in the next few paragraphs.

THE STRENGTH OF MEMORIES

Perhaps it should be stated that the *strength* of a memory is considered here to be a function of the electrical interconnectedness of the component parts of the parent structure. As alluded to earlier, a strong region of a memory would be connected by numerous association linkages, or perhaps by linkages with a higher degree of individual conductivity. If a new memory overlapped such a strong region, it too would be *strong* in this area because of the shared underlying linkages. Weaker structures would, of course, have fewer or less conductive linkages joining the units composing the memory. By the same reasoning, an overlapping new memory should also share these weaker linkages, producing a correspondingly weak area in the new entity. It also seems reasonable to assume that strong regions would be more easily recalled and more durable over time than weaker regions. This arrangement might explain several common observations about memory, as will be discussed.

"MENTAL HOOKS" ON WHICH TO HANG
NEW MEMORIES

It is general knowledge that things that are familiar seem to enter memory more rapidly and easily than information with no prior reference. A list of nonsense syllables or words may be much more difficult to memorize than a sentence that has some meaning for the brain. In fact, students occasionally couple unrelated facts or names with easily remembered sentences to aid memory. The use of mnemonics creates a somewhat artificial form of memory but does illustrate the apparent need to find an appropriate "mental hook" on which to hang new memories. A familiarity with new material (i.e., some reference from prior experience) certainly seems to facilitate the process of learning. This appears generally true for most of the things we learn.

Perhaps the ease or difficulty of learning new material can be explained by the mechanism just proposed for the storage of memories. Recognition and meaningfulness of incoming material would seem to be a function of the degree of matching achieved in the localization process. A high degree of compatibility between structures should yield a greater understanding of the new material. A perception overlapping large portions of existing memories would have a readily available reference in memory, providing it with a hook for easy attachment. Encoding such *familiar* new material would require the formation of fewer new association linkages because of the existing compatibility of the two structures. In contrast, incoming material that does not match significant portions of any existing memory would seem less familiar. Its matched elements might be diffusely spread among many memories and, therefore, understanding from any one entity would be minimal. In other words, meaningfulness in terms of prior experience would be less. Too join the component parts of the structure and establish a new memory would require many more new association linkages, because less existing structure could be utilized. For these reasons, incoming data such as these might appear more difficult to grasp and retain in memory. This may explain the common observation that familiar data are much easier to remember than those that seem alien.

As suggested here, a new memory's strength may at least be partially determined by the strength of the structure to which it corresponds during the storage process. In other words, the strength of a new memory would depend to some degree upon the structures it overlapped. If an incoming perception extensively matched portions of a strong memory, then those regions of the new memory should also be strong because of the shared linkages. If the small memory elements matched by incoming information were diffusely spread among many memories, the resulting structure should be weaker, because there would be little contribution from existing linkages. Thus, completely new information, with little reference in experience, should generally yield weaker memories. As indicated before, it should also be more difficult to store. Memories such as these would also seem more subject to loss through forgetting. This seems to be generally the case. Things that have little meaning for us (i.e., have only marginal reference in experience) seem to form less durable memories. Thus, we hang on to those things that have meaning for us but quickly forget items that appear less significant. The proposed mechanism may provide a biological basis for this phenomenon.

ASSOCIATION LINKAGES AND MEMORY STORAGE

As indicated earlier, learning may involve the strengthening of existing association linkages between the structures destined to become part of the new memory. Alternately, this process might also result from the formation of new synaptic linkages between these elements. In either case, the transmission of energy would be facilitated by these changes, resulting in a more stable and durable structure. It is known that some types of memory formation require a period of consolidation after the initial learning event. This has been well documented by many researchers over the years. If this process is interpreted by electroconvulsive shock (Duncan, 1949) or head trauma (Russell & Nathan, 1946) before it is completed, the new memory will not form. It is presumably during this time that old linkages are strengthened or new ones formed. There is some evidence suggesting that animals exposed to an enriched environment will develop a cortex that is both heavier and thicker than one housed in a less stimulating atmosphere (Bennett, Krech, & Rosenzweig, 1964). It has also been shown by Globus, Rosenzweig, Bennett, and Diamond (1973) that the cortical neurons of rats exposed to an enriched environment develop more dendritic spines, suggesting a greater density of synaptic linkages as a consequence of learning. These findings seem to favor the idea that long-term learning occurs via the growth of new association channels linking the involved structural elements. Perhaps memory formation involves both the enhanced conductance of individual ion channels and an increase in their absolute number. This possibility will now be explored.

The ideas presented here suggest that the conductivity of existing association linkages can be selectively and rapidly modified under many circumstances to initiate new memory storage. The mechanism proposed previously for fantasy formation and the expression of language suggests this possibility. The time required for these mental activities to be accomplished simply seems too brief for the synthesis of new linkages to occur. A change in ionic conduction would seem the only reasonable explanation. This, of course, is probably also true of thinking or any cognitive activity in which old ideas are rapidly combined in new ways. This suggests that a mechanism is available enabling existing association linkages to be selectively opened to rapidly allow the elements of normal thought or fantasy to combine in a coherent but transient way. But, of course, these mental processes do not necessarily lead to lasting memory storage. For the most part, they appear to be ways of manipulating mental entities to accomplish the specific, short-term goals of thinking. It thus appears likely that synaptic linkages can be either acutely modified or increased in absolute number, depending upon the circumstances. The most likely explanation for the presence of both processes is that memory formation begins with the acute modification of existing linkages, as occurs when we combine different ideas in thought. If this process is repeated, consolidation may occur and new linkage growth may be stimulated to increase the durability of the memory. The acute modification of existing connections may allow thoughts to be retained briefly in memory, whereas the formation of new linkages may produce longer term memory.

LONG-TERM POTENTIATION

Experimental work was presented earlier, suggesting that learning and its storage in long-term memory may be the consequence of new synaptic growth occurring over time. Evidence also indicates that existing synaptic connections may be rapidly modified in response to neural activity. In 1973, Bliss and Lomo found that a brief pulse of electrical activity administered to a neural pathway in the hippocampus produced an increase in synaptic strength. This increase in electrical conductance was found to last for hours or even weeks in some situations. This phenomenon is referred to as *long-term potentiation* and is considered to be direct confirmation of Hebb's original postulate. Perhaps this effect or some variation in nonhippocampal cells is responsible for the rapid modification of synaptic junctions, which seems necessary for the expression of thought and the other forms of cognitive activity described earlier.

MEMORY STORAGE OCCURS IN STAGES

In a recent article entitled "The Biological Basis of Learning and Individuality," Kandel and Hawkins (1992) reviewed data from a number of labs indicating that memory storage in *Aplysia* as well as mammals occurs in stages. This work has shown that the establishment of memory lasting from minutes to hours involves changes in the strength of existing synaptic linkages. Such short-term changes are mediated by chemical changes, which are a consequence of current flow through neural pathways. Over time, longer term changes occur, involving the activation of genes and the subsequent generation of new protein and additional synaptic connections. These experimental data support the conception of memory presented in the previous paragraphs of this work.

FACTORS PRODUCING MEMORY ACTIVATION

As indicated, for any large GMC or fresh memory to be activated, it must receive sufficient stimulation from its individual component parts. In other words, the degree of overlap it experiences during the matching process must be significant. This may, however, only be one factor that influences the amount of stimulation received by a complex. In some cases, extensive overlap does not appear necessary to produce complete activation of a large memory. For example, it is common for freshly stored memories to be recalled easily, with only a minimum number of cues from the environment. In contrast, an older memory may require much more prompting for full recall. The face of someone we met yesterday may trigger immediate recall of the entire meeting. Six months later, this might not be sufficient. Several cues in addition to the face might be necessary for full recall. The additional cues required for activation of the older memory suggest a need for greater overlapping of the parent memory (i.e., the need for more component GMCs to be matched). This would seem to indicate that the degree to which a memory is overlapped may not be the only factor in the amount of stimulation generated.

The explanation for these observations may lie in the relative strengths of the involved association linkages. As indicated earlier, this may be a function of the conductivity of individual synaptic connections, or perhaps the overall number of such linkages may determine the amount of energy transmitted. In either case, we can speculate that the synaptic connections holding fresh memories together may be more open and capable of conduction than those of older structures that have faded through disuse. An older complex might be viewed as having more resistance in its connecting linkages. A small, activated component of such a unit would therefore be less capable of conducting neurotransmission to its other associations within the larger structure. In essence, the spread of electrical stimulation would generally be slower and less efficient because of the higher resistance. The opposite would be true of fresh memories. A small, activated component might easily conduct stimulation to the other associated units of the larger complex. It would therefore require fewer small component memories or GMCs to fully activate a fresh complex than an older one. The number of component units necessary to fully stimulate a larger structure would therefore appear to be a function of the age and usage received by the involved memory. The absolute amount of stimulation required may ultimately be dependent upon the relative conductivity of the association linkages involved.

Perhaps a hypothetical example might help to further characterize the factors influencing memory localization. As discussed, any small

GMC may be a functional part of many larger memories or GMCs. In this example, let us assume that such a GMC is a component part of 100 larger entities, each containing an average of 10 smaller GMCs like itself. Let us further assume that of the 100 larger entities, 1 is new (i.e., only 1 of the larger parent structures is a fresh memory). Its association linkages should therefore have less resistance and conduct electrical stimulation more easily than the other 99. When a small GMC is matched by incoming data and activated, the high relative conductivity of the fresh complex may allow all of the other 9 associations of the parent structure to be activated. The overlapping and activation of this single GMC would therefore result in the whole complex receiving stimulation. In contrast, this GMC may activate only 2 or 3 associations in each of the remaining 99 larger complexes. The apparent resistance of their connecting linkages would slow the spread of stimulation in these complexes, preventing their full activation. Each of these would therefore be only partially triggered. The fresh entity would thus be more extensively activated and be fired as a unit, producing its entry into consciousness. The other larger complexes would not fire as intact units, because they experienced less overall stimulation. This example is, of course, consistent with the observation that fresher memories are usually more easily recalled than older ones. In this way, current aspects of life may be maintained in the forefront of thought.

In the preceding hypothetical example, only one GMC was necessary to activate the larger memory because of the strength of its new association linkages. Unfortunately things are probably not this simple in most cases. The situation becomes much more complicated if we assume that there are several new memories in the group, rather than just one. In addition, some of the older memories may still have strong association linkages because of their frequent usage. In such cases, a single GMC may not be sufficient to distinguish a larger entity. Several small GMCs might thus be required. Ultimately, the total amount of stimulation received and the amount of resistant present will determine which large complex is activated. The microstructure of the human brain, with its complex array of converging and diverging fibers, would seem well suited to modulate a system of this potential complexity.

THE "REVEREND"

Our intake of data from the world is usually very rapid and continuous. Identifying individual cues from the environment and correctly pairing them with evoked mental responses are often very difficult under normal conditions. Even so, the careful observer can occasionally catch glimpses of this fleeting phenomenon at work. The following story is an example that provides some insight into memory localization and recall. On a recent evening, a former associate of mine attended a jazz concert performed by a group of amateur musicians from the local community. He immediately recognized the bass fiddle player as someone he had met or seen before. This musician's face was distinctive and familiar, but my associate could recall no details of their prior association. This is a common situation that we have all encountered at one time or another. A face may be recognized as familiar, but it cannot be *placed* in memory. At the end of the concert, the musicians were introduced separately. The fiddle player was initially addressed as "the reverend." At that very instant, my friend recalled his prior relationship with this musician. This man, the pastor of a local church, had visited with his family in their home some 8 weeks earlier. This had been my friend's only contact with this individual, and therefore, his only memory from experience. Upon hearing the word *reverend,* the entire large memory of this prior meeting was triggered into consciousness.

It appears that localization of this memory required two cues from the environment. Both the image of the man's face and the word *reverend* seemed necessary for recognition. Obviously, the image of the face triggered some vague recall of a prior association but was not sufficient to activate the entire memory. In the absence of the face acting as a stimulating cue, it seems unlikely that the word alone would have produced any recall. The word *reverend* is represented in memory as a GMC, and as such, would be present in many large memories. Its lack of specificity in the absence of other cues would make localization of any single memory difficult. In contrast, the memory of the face was specific for a single past memory. Without reinforcement during the 8 weeks since the meeting, it had undergone sufficient deterioration that alone it could not trigger its reference memory. If the concert had occurred shortly after the initial meeting, it would have been stable enough by itself for full localization and recall of the memory of the meeting. In this example, both a partially faded fresh memory and a GMC were required to produce recall. Neither alone would have had the structural strength or specificity to accomplish this. In this unique situation, the two cues necessary to identify the reference memory were separated in time by approximately 1 hour and therefore presented as separate events that could be clearly identified. If the bass fiddle player had been introduced at the start of the concert, the two necessary cues would have been closely paired and not recognized as separate. The brain would have been unaware that these two separate components were both necessary for recognition of the memory. The separation of these events in time seems to provide us with valuable insight into the processes involved.

The previous example also demonstrates several principles discussed earlier. The memory in question was localized only because of the uniqueness of the two cues involved. In the great volume of memories stored within my friend's brain, these two smaller memories were components of only the one reference memory. This memory was specified because the two cues necessary for recall occurred nowhere else together. In this case, they provided sufficient stimulating energy to activate the original memory. This seems to be the basic principle underlying localization. GMCs or fresh memories are activated by incoming data until a unique combination specifying only a single larger memory is achieved. Such a localized memory would, of course, receive more

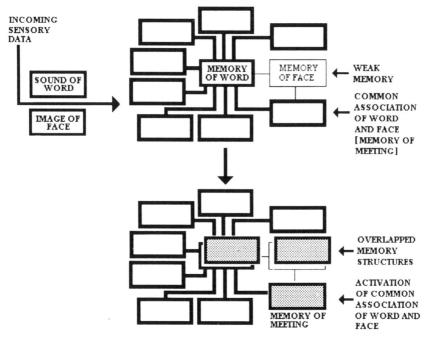

Figure 3.2 In this figure, squares and rectangles represent memories, which may contain many neurons. The symbol for the face was drawn in thin black lines to indicate that it has faded somewhat. In the lower part of the figure, the sound of the word *reverend* and the image of his face match and overlap corresponding structures in memory storage. In combination, these two entities provide enough energy for activation of their common associations, which, upon activation, specify for the brain their relationship from prior experience. In this case, the memory of the meeting is activated.

stimulating energy than other entities. In some way, this would designate the most closely matched structure for the brain.

Perhaps, at this point, it would be helpful to summarize "the reverend" example and the conclusions that were drawn. The sequence of events suggests that the memory of the meeting was triggered by two cues. It is assumed that the word *reverend* is represented in memory by a small GMC and, as such, is probably a component of many larger GMCs and memories. Its localization would produce some activation in all these larger entities, including the memory of the meeting with the pastor. This, however, was not sufficient by itself to trigger any of these parent complexes. In contrast, the memory of the face was specific and was associated only with the memory of the meeting. By itself, the image of the musician was also insufficient to trigger the larger memory, because it had weakened through disuse. In combination, there was apparently enough neurotransmission to activate the entire larger complex. Because only one larger memory contained this unique combination of cues, it received enough stimulation to trigger the full parent memory. "The reverend" example is illustrated in Figure 3.2.

VISUALIZING THE LOCALIZATION PROCESS

If we could visualize the localization process during the intake of sensory data, we might see multiple streaks of neurotransmission crisscrossing each other within the brain. Each would arise as a GMC was activated and its energy transmitted to its associations. In some places, several of these streaks would cross, designating larger complexes that contained several of the smaller GMCs linked in association. The point of maximum intersection would designate the structure most closely corresponding to the incoming data. As indicated, the absolute amount of stimulation received by this identified complex would probably be a balance of the total number of components activated and the relative strengths of their connecting linkages. The large structure most closely matching the incoming perception would thus be localized.

CHAPTER OVERVIEW

The system of memory storage described would depend upon the generation of numerous small memory units that could combine in various ways to create larger memories. These small units of memory would be composed of discrete neural patterns created through specific modifications in the conductance of association linkages. Such patterns would originally be created in the neurons of the sensory perception areas in response to incoming information. To facilitate longer term storage, these patterns would be transferred to the memory storage regions, where they would be duplicated. If reinforced, these newly established patterns would become more durable. Larger memories would be created by streams of such data over time. Relationships between such information would be expressed by the generation of association linkages. Large complexes of interrelated data, strung together to reflect their association in experience, would be common and numerous. The localization of memories would follow the same sequence of steps used to initially store them. Their component pieces would be matched and overlapped by incoming data until sufficient energy was received for activation. The energy generated in this process would be passed on to any associated memories, which would be activated and reenter the sensory perception areas to define the original perception. The interpretation of new data would thus be expressed in terms already familiar to the brain. This will be dealt with further in the next chapter.

4

Consciousness

Consciousness is perhaps the greatest mystery of the human brain. Through the ages, volumes have been written in an effort to comprehend this elusive and fascinating aspect of mental activity. Perhaps it can most simply be viewed as a state of perceptual awareness, although philosophical definitions are often more complex. For most people, consciousness is synonymous with self. It is often considered to be the very seat of human existence and individuality. Through its portals, we witness the passage of our own inner thoughts and the world around us. It is the center of each individual's personal universe and the reference by which we define our very existence. It is the interface between the deeper reaches of the brain and the external world.

We experience consciousness as an awareness of verbal thoughts, memories, sensory data, and emotion. Although this seems self-evident, Klinger and Cox (1987–1988) have experimentally studied this subject. In their work, 1,400 thought samples were taken over time from 29 subjects and analyzed. These authors found that 73% of thought contained some interior verbal commentary and 67% had some degree of visual imagery. Unfortunately, these subjects were not questioned about their affective reactions during thought.

The aforementioned elements of thought are familiar parts of our inner conscious world. Their expression is so spontaneous and natural that we rarely question their origin. Thoughts just seem to flow through the brain, without obvious composition or effort. If we carefully examine this phenomenon, it appears that much of what is commonly attributed to consciousness actually originates out of direct awareness. Although we see our thoughts, their origin and formulation are largely hidden from view. Full sentences, expressing our feelings, commenting on our activities or current situations, seem to emerge spontaneously from the brain for our consideration. Obviously, at least part of what we observe in consciousness arises at a deeper level. Through the awareness of consciousness, we bear witness to an almost continuous stream of mental activity. We are in some way both observers and directors of this familiar scenario.

STIMULUS–RESPONSE MODEL OF CONSCIOUSNESS

Chains of related thoughts flow from our brains when we think. The process appears to be one of stimulus and response. Every inwardly spoken sentence or thought seems to serve as a focal point initiating the next. In sequence, each appears to pivot on the one just preceding, stimulating a new response. Ideas progress from one to the next in related fashion, suggesting that thought has a basic form of organization. It seems probable that the physical association of related memories may form the underlying basis for this phenomenon. In such an arrangement, thoughts would arise from the flow of neurotransmission through associated networks of memories. The sequential activation of electrically linked neural circuits might thus be responsible for the connectedness observed in thought. These ideas suggest that new thoughts arise from the associations of memories that were used to generate earlier thoughts. In other words, such associations might provide the building blocks necessary for the composition of additional thoughts.

CONVERSATION AS AN EXTENSION OF CONSCIOUSNESS

In many ways, thinking resembles normal conversation. Spoken sentences, like thoughts, seem linked in association and therefore flow from one subject to another in a harmonious, related manner. This can be easily observed in everyday conversation. Comments made by a speaker seem to function like thoughts, in that they stimulate additional mental activity in the listener. These incoming data are processed by the brain, resulting in an appropriate remark or interpretation, which can then be expressed verbally or in thought. In fact, sentences spoken in conversation seem to be just an external projection of normal thought. In this way, conversation seems to follow the same stimulus–response model proposed for thought. It is not difficult to imagine that both processes originate in the unconscious interpretive areas of the brain from the same basic mechanism.

THE FLOW OF THOUGHT IN CONSCIOUSNESS

The interpretive phase of thought has been partially characterized in the preceding section. This process begins with a stimulus, which can be a spoken sentence, a sensory perception, or a preceding thought. Beginning in the sensory perception areas, this stimulus is transmitted to memory storage, where the interpretative process begins. Through comparative matching, GMCs (generalized memory complexes), or individual memories, are located and overlapped electrically in appropriate areas by incoming stimuli. In other words, memory structures that are similar to the incoming perception are identified and activated during this process. As a consequence, associated memories are activated,

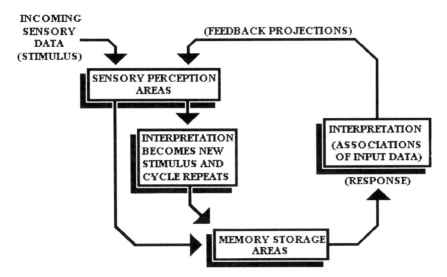

Figure 4.1 Incoming data and/or thoughts are registered in appropriate sensory cortices before traveling on to memory storage areas, where localization and matching of corresponding structures occur. As a result of this, associated memories are activated, which provide an interpretation for the incoming information. Through feedback projections, this interpretation, which now functions as a new stimulus, is channeled back through the appropriate sensory cortices and the process is repeated, resulting in the production of a new thought (interpretation). It is proposed that consciousness arises as a consequence of this cyclic process.

PART A

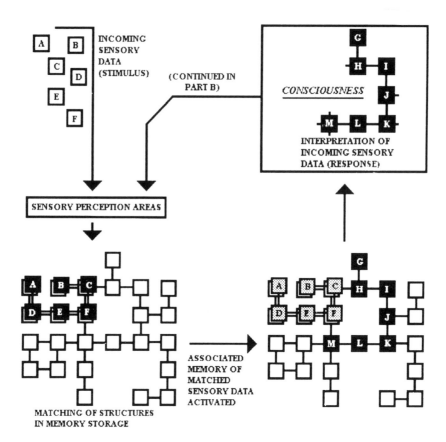

Figure 4.2a This figure illustrates how the sequential activation of electrically linked memories might lead to associated thought. In the upper-left corner of this figure, a sensory perception, composed of A–F, enters the brain and matches corresponding structures in memory storage. In sequence, its associations, G–M, are activated and perceived in consciousness as an interpretation for the original perception. This memory then travels back to the appropriate sensory perception areas, and the process continues in part b of this figure.

PART B

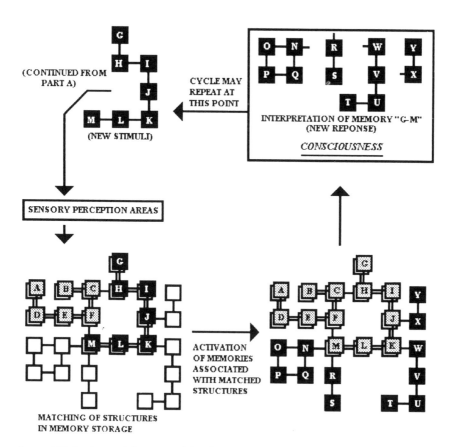

Figure 4.2b In the top-left corner of this figure, the first interpretation from part a passes through the sensory perception area and overlaps corresponding structures in memory storage. This produces the sequential activation of associated memories, which serve as the second interpretation (the "interpretation" for the first interpretation). These activated memories are labeled O–Q, R–S, T–W and X–Y. At this point, they may be combined with each other in new ways or combined with entities already in short-term memory (from previous rounds of thought) to produce unique stimuli that can again undergo interpretation. It is proposed that this process can continue to produce long chains of related thought.

which enter consciousness and provide interpretation for the incoming data. New information can thus be understood because of its similarity to older knowledge previously stored in memory. This process is illustrated in the following two figures. In Figure 4.1, the cyclic flow of thought, as described here, is depicted; in Figures 4.2a and 4.2b, the movement of thought from one associated memory to the next is illustrated.

INTERPRETATIONS ARE THE PRODUCT OF PRIOR EXPERIENCE

The many memories and GMCs stored in the brain do not exist alone. Each has numerous other such entities linked in association, as established through experience. When a GMC or memory is matched to an incoming perception during the localization process, any memories held in association by the identified entities also receive energy and are activated. Such associations enter consciousness and provide understanding for the incoming perception. In other words, new information is defined in the same terms used for the older data, to which it corresponds. During the processing of new information, many individual memories and GMCs may cumulatively contribute something to the overall meaning through the activation of their associative memories. The final interpretation derived in this way would ultimately be the product of prior experience. It would represent a response to the original stimulus and might often be expressed as a subsequent sentence or thought.

CONSCIOUSNESS IN PREVERBAL MAN

In preverbal man, this response was probably a combination of evoked memories and emotion. At this point, words were not available as a form of mental communication. In many animals of today, a similar form of consciousness may still exist. When a memory or GMC is activated, its associations, as well as any linked emotion, are released and enter consciousness. As will be discussed in a later chapter, emotions also seem to function as associations of memories and are sensed when the memory is activated. These entities, in combination with sensory memories, probably serve as nonverbal interpretations for matched perceptions. Through the localization process, the organism may activate visual or other sensory memories of similar past situations, which may serve as literal translations for the new data. Fear, anger, pleasure, or any combination of emotions linked in association with the activated memories may also be experienced. Their release would, of course, constitute an emotional interpretation for the present situation. Prior knowledge is therefore used to impart meaning. Memories of prior experience may thus provide an emotional and literal understanding for new situations through the matching process.

EMOTIONS IN CONSCIOUSNESS

Some emotions released during the interpretation process may produce an autonomic response in the body, whereas others may be less intense and only convey a subtle mental awareness. We may sense that the situation is understood or perhaps confusing. We may experience surprise, satisfaction, or any number of other emotional states that inform us of the situation at hand. Emotions, therefore, seem to serve as a form of communication between the unconscious interpretative areas of the brain and the awareness we know as consciousness. They impart meaning to those memories activated during the interpretation phase and, in turn, to the general situation under consideration. The emotion we experience from any given situation is a blend of all those released during the interpretative process. This is probably a natural consequence of the mixing of GMCs and memories to match incoming data. Numerous such entities may be utilized to define any given situation, and each may release emotion, which contributes something to the overall emotional interpretation. In this way, the emotional response is custom-tailored to the perception in question. In primitive man, everything was probably sensed and understood through the release of emotion and nonverbal memories. All situations were judged by the emotion imparted during interpretation. This will be discussed in more detail in a later section on emotion.

Perhaps a simple example of learned animal behavior might illustrate the process by which emotions provide interpretation for memories. In experiments performed in 1972, Rizley and Rescorla conditioned rats by pairing a sound with a subsequent light in repetitive training sessions. Later, when exposed to the sound, there was no change in behavior or obvious emotional release. In further training sessions, these rats were exposed to a light followed by a painful electrical shock. These rats now reacted quite differently when exposed to the original sound. When challenged, their movement stopped, and they crouched in anticipation of the shock. They clearly appeared to be reacting with fear to the upcoming shock. In some way, they had come to associate the sound with the shock, despite the fact that these events had never been directly paired in experience. According to the hypothesis presented here, the memories of the sound and the light became associated through repetition during the training sessions. The synaptic linkages joining the two GMCs corresponding to these sensory perceptions became more open, expediting neurotransmission. In other words, their electrical connectivity had strengthened so that when the memory of the sound was activated, the memory of the light was also triggered as an associated memory. In subsequent conditioning, the light and the shock became paired in a similar way. Through this process, both pairs of events became sequentially linked. An electrical pathway was created, joining the initial sound with the light and on to the shock. When the animal experienced the sound, this triggered memories of the light and then the shock. It was thus able to anticipate both future events, and the associated emotion was released, leading to the interpretation that the situation was potentially dangerous. This was evident by the fear reaction that occurred before the actual shock.

STRUCTURE OF ASSOCIATIVE MEMORY

In the previous example, a large memory seems to have arisen through the combination of three smaller components. As suggested before, basic units of memory probably grow into larger complexes in this way, reflecting new learning. The small constituents of such a memory may also be parts of many other functioning memories, or larger GMCs. Each larger complex would be characterized by a specific pattern of neurotransmission, defining it as a separate and individual entity. The small elements composing such a structure might each have a separate meaning when not linked in combination. As an electrically joined unit, such individual pieces would have a cumulative meaning unique to the structure as a whole. In this case, the three small units of memory combined to form a larger complex with a specific and frightening meaning for the rat. Such a connotation would not have been possible from the individual components considered separately.

When a memory is initially stored, a specific path of neurotransmission is probably established, linking its associated elements. If not reinforced, the strength of this path may deteriorate over time. In the previous example, the sound alone was sufficient to produce activation of the fresh memory, as indicated by the animals' response. Over time and without reinforcement, some forgetting of the memory would be expected. Presumably, the association linkages joining the components of this memory would undergo some deterioration in electrical conductance, producing reduced recall. At this later point, it might require both the sound and light to activate the overall memory and to recall the shock. This may be a general principal of most memories. As they age and fade through disuse, more cues from the environment seem to be required to produce recall. This was discussed in the last chapter.

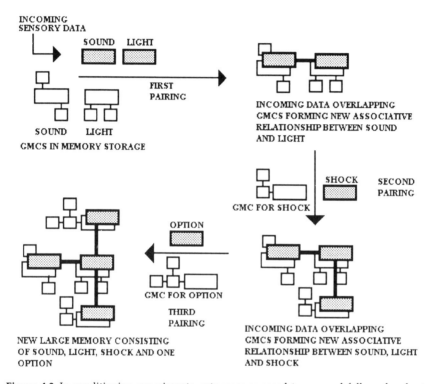

Figure 4.3 In conditioning experiments, rats were exposed to a sound followed a short time later by a light. Each of these sensory perceptions entered memory storage and were electrically overlapped with their appropriate GMC. Through repetition, these memories became linked in association (i.e., their synaptic connections became more open to neurotransmission). In subsequent training sessions, the light was paired with a painful shock. In the same way, a path of neurotransmission was also opened between these two memories. At this point, these three memories were electrically connected, creating a larger unit functioning as a single entity. When challenged with a sound, a conditioned rat could anticipate the shock, even though these two events had never been paired directly in experience. Because of their electrical connectivity, activation of the sound's memory led to that of the light and on to the shock. When an option was created for the rat, its memory became associated with the light, and a branch point was created. Now, exposure to the sound stimulated both the memory of the shock and its option to be activated. The rat could now predict these future events and the consequences of any chosen action.

In this specific example, the rat has no way to avoid the shock once the sequence has begun. It might properly interpret its predicament but be unable to alter its fate. Let us suppose that it were given an option by having a portion of its cage insulated from electrical shock. Over time, it would learn that by moving to this area when the sound occurred, it could avoid the shock as well as the anticipatory anxiety and fear. Through this process the memory specifying the situation would be modified by the acquisition of an additional part. The memory of the new option would become linked in association with the main body of the GMC, creating a branch point within the structure. Each limb originating at this branch point would lead to the memory of one of the available options. The rat would now realize that at least two possibilities existed each time it heard the sound. It could remain on the grid and receive the shock, or move to the insulated area and thus avoid this unpleasant physical sensation. As it experiences the visual memory of each option, the corresponding associated emotion would be released. Each visual image would be interpreted in this way to provide it with the information to make a decision and act. The choice would be clear, and it would move to the insulated portion of the cage. If further options were added, the GMC would acquire more branch points, and the process leading to a final decision would become more complex. Presumably the emotion associated with each choice would guide any final decision. In this way, emotions seem to influence and direct our thoughts and lead to the actions we ultimately choose. This important concept will be discussed later. Figure 4.3 illustrates the neural changes that may have occurred in the rat experiments.

LITERAL AND EMOTIONAL INTERPRETATIONS IN PREVERBAL THINKING

In the modern human brain, interpretations are expressed by a mixture of entities. Consciousness is experienced as silently spoken words mixed with memories of sensory data. There is always a background emotional tone (mood), which may become dominant during the evaluation of emotionally charged situations. In preverbal man, all memories were probably representations of the physical world as perceived through the senses. Visual images were mixed with memories of sounds, smells, and other directly observable data. In essence, the external world was recorded internally by the creation of specific neural patterns that could be activated for future reference. Thinking was simple and probably consisted of the recall and recombination of relevant memories and associated emotion in response to sensory challenges. Interpretations of incoming data were thus a combination of literal and emotional elements.

The ability to recombine visual images from memory in different ways is a form of *generativity*. This term refers to a general ability or property, which, according to theory, originally arose as a unique cognitive style in the human left brain, for the control of motor skill, or praxis (Corballis, 1989). It has been postulated that image generativity involves breaking visual imagery into elementary geometric components, or *geons*, which can be recombined and manipulated (Kosslyn, 1987). It is assumed this is largely a function of the left hemisphere, since the left brain seems more skilled than the right at breaking stimuli down into categorical elements that can be recombined to form novel images (Farah, 1984; Kosslyn, 1988). Because this process allows the brain to organize basic units of information into multipart representations, generativity can be considered to be an analytic as well as combinatorial skill. This general cognitive style may have facilitated early tool building and, through its ability to recombine phonemes and words, language may have evolved. It is proposed that preverbal thought in early man may have employed generativity to produce recombinations of visual images. Through the narrative chains produced in this way, it should have been possible to envision and manipulate events stored in memory to produce a form of thinking independent of spoken language. As will be explained in the next chapter, emotion arising from this recombination of such mental entities may have produced guidance for this primitive form of cognition.

EVOLUTION OF ASSOCIATED LANGUAGE

Over time, language developed. We can speculate that the memories of verbal sounds became electrically linked through association with the mental representations of objects in the environment. In this way, words were created and given meaning by their associated memory of the physical world. The usage of various words was passed from one person to another by mimicking these sounds, which had become associated with things being named. This is known as onomatopoeia, which literally means "the making of a word." The earliest words probably symbolized single objects in the environment. Over time, words came to define various simple relationships observed in nature. Eventually, complex relationships involving many objects became linked through association to form concepts. We can imagine that the GMC for a word or concept might have at its core a basic neural structure representing the memory of the sound. This would be the site where perceptions would be electrically matched. In turn, this would be synaptically connected to one or more memories defining the word or concept as a whole. These, of course, would be associations of the memory representing the sound. A word matched through the localization process would in turn activate its defining memories. This might be a single mental representation of an object or perhaps a number of memories defining a concept. This arrangement may have made it possible to link words together to concisely describe complex mental pictures of the world. A shorthand method of information exchange between people had evolved. Minds became linked through verbal communication, enabling a sharing of knowledge and an enormous expansion of each individual's mental database. This single evolutionary development may explain humankind's dominance in the animal kingdom.

INTERPRETATION OF LANGUAGE

When we hear spoken language, it probably enters the brain and is interpreted like any other auditory perception. Each word is matched to its appropriate GMC through the localization process. This structure contains the memory of the word and is electrically linked to the object or concept to which it has become associated through usage. The localization of the GMC activates this meaning, which enters consciousness and defines the word for the brain. Each word of a sentence may be sequentially localized and activated in this manner, providing an overall meaning for the group of words. It should be emphasized that this is probably the exact process that occurs when nonverbal sensory perceptions are interpreted. In each case, component GMCs are overlapped and activated by incoming data to yield an interpretation that is the sum of the individual parts. When language is used, words are localized and converted into their sensory counterparts, which can be directly understood by the brain. When nonverbal events are involved, interpretation occurs without the need for this extra verbal-translation step. It would thus appear that language may have evolved as an extension of a mechanism already in place. Because this process occurs in the unconscious interpretative area, it is out of normal awareness. Through this process of translation, incoming words paint an almost instantaneous picture, which allows us to understand spoken language.

PURPOSE OF INTERPRETATION

The *purpose* of interpretation is to understand sensory input and thought. All incoming data are subjected to the comparative matching process so that meaning can be derived from prior experience. In many cases, this phase of thought yields more than just a basic understanding. For example, predictions of future events can be made, based upon the outcome of similar past circumstances. This was clearly illustrated in the rat experiments in which animals learned to anticipate a shock. Many situations may be at least partially new, and no exact match with prior experience can be made. Some understanding may occur by combining several prior similar situations. This might be accomplished by the over-lapping of various regions of the incoming perception with several GMCs, or fresh memories that correspond structurally. This mixed form of interpretation would allow the brain to combine prior knowledge to extract meaning, as discussed previously. If sufficient overlap could be achieved, some understanding would seem possible. Obviously, the more a situation deviates from past experience, the poorer will be the understanding and any prediction made. Even so, this is not uncommon in life. We often guess at things because of inadequate knowledge. By ex-tracting information from several past situations, mixed interpretations would seem possible. In this way, some degree of understanding can be derived for any event that lacks exact corresponding prior experience. Considering the vast number of ways the elements of life can be com-bined, a system such as this would seem essential.

INTERPRETATION OCCURS AT AN UNCONSCIOUS LEVEL

As indicated before, interpretations are made at an unconscious level. In the primitive brain, the results of this process were probably expressed in consciousness through the recall of sensory data and emotion. In modern man, thoughts are largely verbal but can still be mixed with vi-sual images or other sensory memories. Emotion is still an important part of the interpretation process. Language has largely replaced sen-sory memories in consciousness, because it is the medium of communi-cation with others. It also provides a more precise way of expressing thought than possible with sensory memories. The conversion of words into their corresponding nonverbal associations during interpretation has already been discussed. It seems probable that conclusions from this process are then converted back into language through a reverse-translation process prior to entering consciousness. In this way, ideas are expressed in a form that can be directly communicated to others if desired, or recycled through the brain as thoughts.

THINKING AS A CYCLIC PROCESS

It is postulated here that thinking is a cyclic process. Thoughts expressed in words leave the interpretative portions of the brain and are channeled into the sensory perception areas. At this point, they join the pathway taken by all incoming sensory data. In the same way that information from the senses becomes conscious, these verbal data generated during the interpretative process probably also enter active awareness. Such data are then passed back into the interpretive areas, where they are evaluated again and understood. Through this closed, cyclic loop, our unconscious thoughts become known to the brain. We see our thoughts as we do any incoming sensory perception, but through the interpretative process, they are understood and recognized as being of internal origin. This hypothesis suggests that thoughts are generated by the unconscious evaluation of data that arise from external perception or previous thought. Such information is then cycled through the perception and interpretative areas, where conscious understanding is achieved. Only at this point do we become aware of their content. It is as if one portion of the brain is speaking to another.

VISUAL PERCEPTIONS AND CONSCIOUSNESS

In 1970, Segal and Fusella produced evidence that competition exists between a visual image held in consciousness and a simultaneous incoming visual perception. Onto a translucent screen they projected a white spot whose luminosity could be varied. Subjects were asked to watch the screen and to imagine a tree. At the same time, the luminosity of the white spot was increased gradually until the subject reported seeing it. Control groups were told to imagine a sound, such as the ringing of a telephone, or to make their minds blank. Surprisingly, the intensity needed for perception of the light was much greater in the subjects imagining the tree, as compared to either control group. In other words, competition existed between the incoming visual perception and the internally generated mental image. In contrast, the auditory memory produced no competition with the visual perception. One interpretation of these data is that mental images, as suggested here, pass through the visual cortex to achieve awareness in the brain. A simultaneous, incoming visual perception would compete for the same circuitry producing the effects observed. In contrast, the auditory memory did not interfere with visual perception, because it entered consciousness via the auditory cortex.

In another study by Antrobus, Singer, Goldstein, and Fortgang (1970), complementary results were obtained. Subjects were asked to do signal-detection tasks involving either visual or auditory stimuli. It was found that visual tasks interfered with daydreams composed of visual images more than those that were auditory in content. The opposite results were found when auditory tasks were performed (i.e., auditory daydreams were decreased in comparison to those with a visual content). These data again support the contention that memories of various sensory modalities pass through their respective cortices to gain awareness in the brain. Further evidence for this will be presented later in this chapter, when the phenomenon of blindsight is considered.

Once thoughts enter consciousness, they continue to be processed as any incoming sensory perception. They are subjected to the same localization and matching process, and undergo reinterpretation. Any new conclusions that result are again expressed as words or feelings and cycled back into consciousness. As indicated before, each thought seems to act as a stimulus, producing a subsequent thought as the response. This cycle may be repeated over and over many times, producing long chains of thought. This is probably the essence of thinking as we know it.

THINKING ALOUD

The cyclic nature of thought can perhaps be more easily visualized by observing ourselves thinking aloud. In this practice, thoughts are projected externally in speech. Almost everyone talks to him- or herself from time to time. This practice is common and may help with concentration in distracting situations. Thoughts arising from the interpretative area of the brain leave the mouth as speech. There is no prior conscious awareness of what is to be expressed. Only when the words are heard through the ears do we sense their content and meaning. The *inner voice* we associate with thinking has been projected as speech, rather than as internal thought. In this process, the brain actually appears to be talking to itself. There is a speaker and listener, as occurs in conversation. Thought leaves one region of the brain and is only appreciated when it enters a second area. From time to time, we all say things we regret. We often respond by wondering, "Why would I say something like that?" Again this reflects the unknown nature of thought prior to its perception and interpretation. Thoughts that cycle in this manner lead to new thoughts, and the process continues. By examining the way we think out loud, this cyclic nature becomes more obvious. It also demonstrates the relationship between thinking and conversation. Both processes can be described by a stimulus–response model that sequentially drives the cyclic movement of information.

THOUGHTS AS INTERPRETATIONS
OF PRIOR THOUGHTS

When a cycling thought enters the interpretative area, it acts as a stimulus for additional mental activity. A new thought, which is related through association to the first, is produced. It gains conscious awareness after passing through the sensory perception areas and undergoing reinterpretation. At this point, it becomes a stimulus and the cycle repeats itself. In this way, new thoughts may be produced in chainlike fashion. As indicated before, each thought entering the interpretative area undergoes comparative matching where corresponding GMCs or fresh memories are identified. These, in turn, trigger their associated memories and emotion to provide meaning. It is from these memories that new thoughts originate. They are, in fact, an interpretation of the previous thought derived from the associated memories that are activated in this process. A given stimulus may trigger a number of previously unrelated GMCs and fresh memories. These produce an overall interpretation based upon their mixed combination. A new thought thus reflects any conclusions arising in this way. Every new thought can therefore be considered to be an interpretation of a prior thought acting as a stimulus. In a like manner, any emotions released from these activated memories combine to yield an additional interpretation. A thought's meaning is thus expressed verbally as well as emotionally.

CYCLIC CONSCIOUSNESS PRODUCES
ASSOCIATED THOUGHT

This proposed model for cyclic thought provides some insight into the observation that thoughts, as well as spoken sentences, generally follow each other in associated manner. Each interpretation derived in this process is extracted from memories, which are themselves in association with the original stimulus. This is, of course, suggested by the associated coherence that is normally present in speech and thought. A disruption of this process often occurs in psychosis. In some forms of schizophrenia, thought form is so disorganized that normal coherence is lost. Sentences unrelated in content are strung together to produce a meaningless monologue to the listener. This illustrates the normal importance of associated thought and speech. This process occurs so naturally that it often goes unnoticed in routine conversation. Without it, thought and speech would not be possible as we know it. Obviously there must be some basic underlying mechanism in mental activity to account for it. The model proposed here seems to explain this phenomenon.

STORING AND RECALLING AN ASSOCIATED MEMORY

Perhaps at this point, a specific example might help to illustrate the principles of mental activity proposed in this chapter. Let us assume that you are in need of a new chair and have decided to visit a local furniture store. As you walk through this establishment, every type of furniture imaginable seems to be present. There are lamps, chairs, beds, tables, couches, and so forth. The visual perception of each produces instant recognition. The GMC for each of these items has been located, providing identification from past experience. The specific memory of each item thus identified is stored in overlapped fashion with its corresponding GMC. A new, fresh memory has thus been combined with a cluster of older, generalized memories. Each item processed in this way is linked in association, producing a mental representation of your trip through the store. These memories are also linked with any other sensory perceptions that may have been present. For example, the smell and general appearance of the store, as well as the attitudes of the sales personnel, will be recorded. Each of these quantities is identified and stored in the same way as described for the furniture. In addition to basic identification, the evaluation process may yield other judgments. For example, we may like or dislike certain furniture styles based upon prior standards stored in memory. These judgments are part of each GMC, and are a summary of what we have come to value from past experience. This knowledge may also allow us to assess the appropriateness of each item for our use, its price, and even the quality of service received at the store. Any chair we select will be a complex mixture of these value judgments.

The visit to the store constitutes a large sensory perception, processed bit by bit. Each piece of data is taken in and referenced to prior knowledge to produce a continuous chain of interpretation for our immediate use. This is an ongoing process that also produces a sequential memory of the events as they occur. Specific memories are stored with their corresponding GMCs and linked together in association to record the entire sequence of events as witnessed. These are, in turn, linked to any judgments rendered during the process. Information organized in this way allows recall of memories to follow lines of association. If we later reflect on our visit to the store, one memory will trigger another, and so forth, allowing a coherent recall of events. As indicated before, this is a direct reflection of the cyclic nature of thought. Each memory of an item or event that occurred in the store enters the interpretative area and is matched with its corresponding memory. This, in turn, causes an associated memory to be released into consciousness. The process is repeated, and another association is called up. Each cycle moves the mental focus to another association, allowing the entire memory of the store visit to be recalled a piece at a time, if desired.

COGNITIVE MANIPULATION OF MEMORIES IN THINKING

In the previous example, the interpretation of a large sensory perception was described. Conclusions derived from prior experience were transferred to the present situation to provide meaning and understanding. The search and matching process occurred in response to a continuous flow of information from the senses. This appears to be a common mental process, which allows us to deal with incoming information. But what about the cognitive manipulation of previously stored material, that is, the type of mental activity we usually refer to as thinking? Can we speculate on the process by which existing memories are used to arrive at new conclusions, not apparent through the initial matching procedure?

To examine this question, let us suppose that two seemingly unrelated situations stored in memory are to be examined. Through this process we hope to find relationships not previously seen. Each memory under consideration is large and consists of numerous small GMCs (associations) linked electrically in a way that reflects their relationship in nature. The process is begun when one of the memories is localized and its associations are recalled into consciousness, one by one. This may occur via the cyclic process previously described. In this way, the brain is able to review each part of the large memory representing the situation. Through this process, the details of the memory are called into consciousness, where they will remain in short-term memory for a brief time. Stored in this way, thoughts may linger in the background while others are actively considered. In this manner, they appear to remain readily available for reference if needed. At this point, the memory of the second situation to be compared is called forth, and its component associations are reviewed in the same way. Through this process, each memory's associations are brought together and briefly held in consciousness so they can be examined simultaneously. If associations common to both situations are present, it seems likely that they will be recognized in this manner. Of course, any shared association identified in this way represents a previously unrecognized relationship between the two large memories. Comparison of separate entities in this manner seems possible only because of the brief retention of component pieces provided by short-term memory.

As indicated, an association held jointly by two memories reflects a relationship between these entities. They share a common element and in this way are related. Identification of shared associations would seem to be possible through this comparative process. We can imagine that the brain might frequently shift back and forth between memories to ensure that all associations were recalled and compared. This is probably a common form of cognitive analysis, applicable to many situations. A complex situation may be analyzed in this way by cycling many thoughts through consciousness, looking for previously unrecognized relationships. This seems to be the basic process we use when mulling over a situation we do not understand. Many subtle relationships not initially recognized at the time of memory storage can be realized in this manner. The process described is probably the basis for *deductive reasoning*. Much of our knowledge base is probably acquired in this manner and supplements that from direct observation.

The objective of the process described is to identify common associations held by two or more larger memories. In this way, relationships between them become recognized. An obvious question at this point is why all common associations are not discovered during the initial matching process. This is, after all, a process in which similar or identical structures are identified. To answer this, we must look at what happens during this process. Assume that memory A, already in storage, contains a number of common associations with an incoming perception, which will be stored as memory B. This, of course, indicates that these two entities have some common relationship in nature. During the localization and matching process, these common components will overlap each other. If enough shared components exist between A and B, there will be sufficient matching, so that A will be completely activated when B enters the brain and is stored as a memory. In this case, the relationship between these two entities should be obvious, because A would actually serve as part of the interpretation for B. If, however, there are only a few common associations shared by these two memories, A may only be partially activated by B during the matching process. In other words, B may not sufficiently overlap A to produce its activation as a whole. The activation of A would be limited to those few associations held in common with B. In this case, the relationship between these two larger entities would not be identified at the time B was added to memory storage. Although these few common associations would be overlapped during matching, the failure of A to be totally activated would prevent this relationship from being established at that time. The brain would therefore not fully recognize the relationships between the larger parent structures A and B. The system seems to be designed so that only strongly related events are identified as similar during the initial matching and localization process. More subtle relations would be discovered only through the direct comparison of memories in consciousness, as described earlier.

A SIMILARITY TO STIMULUS GENERALIZATION

It should be noted that the principles described previously are similar to those of *stimulus generalization,* discussed earlier. In other words, memory groups sharing only a few common elements would not be perceived as similar, and the stimulus would not generalize. As the occurrence of common elements becomes greater, the two groups will be seen as more similar, and generalization would occur more frequently. This, of course, suggests that the basic process described here may be the same as stimulus generalization, which has been recognized for many years.

BASIC INTERPRETATIONS FROM INITIAL EVALUATIONS OF DATA

Could there be a biological reason why all relationships are not realized during initial interpretation of new data? We can speculate that the initial matching process was intended to yield only literal and straightforward interpretations. In many cases, incoming data would need to be rapidly processed so that the matters at hand could be dealt with expeditiously. For this reason, there would need to be a good match between data to be evaluated and existing memories. If poor matches were allowed, interpretations might be ambiguous and perhaps confusing. This could not be tolerated in a situation in which some immediate action might be required. Survival, in many cases, depends upon a clear and accurate analysis of the immediate situation. This would seem to be an important aspect of any initial evaluation of data and may be why all relationships are not initially seen.

CONCRETE AND ABSTRACT THINKING

The initial interpretative process described previously probably recognizes only gross similarities between things and may be the basis for what is commonly referred to as *concrete thinking*. Most children and adults with some forms of mental illness employ this as their main form of information processing. In contrast, cognitive analysis allows more subtle relationships between things to be determined. Ideas related by only a few associations held in common may be identified by the mechanism proposed earlier. Through this form of analysis, unseen relationships may be discovered. This process is frequently used in research, and is probably the basis for *abstract thinking*. Because it identifies relationships that can be very subtle, it is obviously not well suited for initial evaluations of data in which rapid, concrete judgments are usually necessary.

IDENTIFICATION OF COMMON ASSOCIATIONS

Examples of thinking utilizing the type of *cognitive reflection* described here are common. We frequently attempt to link ideas or find relationships between things that have no obvious connection in experience. Consider the following situation: Bipolar mood disorder is a psychiatric illness characterized by periodic cycles in mood. Patients may exhibit profound depression that alternates over time with manic episodes. The biological basis for this is unknown. Hormonal secretion is also a phenomenon that seems cyclic in nature. For example, the pituitary gland releases substances that cause the adrenal glands to secrete cortisone. Peak levels are detected in the morning at the time of waking and progressively decrease throughout the day. The lowest levels are found at bedtime. This is a cyclic process that seems to have been established through millennia of dark–light cycles corresponding to sleeping–waking periods. Bipolar mood disorder and hormone secretion are two basically dissimilar concepts but are related by the common fact that both are cyclic in nature. This one fact expresses a relationship between them and therefore represents a common association shared by each. Could this illness be related to the cyclic secretion of one or more hormones, or could they both be related to some underlying biological clock? By employing cognitive analysis, the cyclic nature of both processes can be recognized and understood as an element common to both large concepts. In other words, an association common to both *A* and *B* has been discovered through cognitive processing of each memory. It is unlikely that this relationship would have been detected during the initial matching process, because the two bodies of knowledge are so basically dissimilar. Obviously, some process must be in place to allow them to be compared at a later time. This type of cognitive analysis is probably employed in virtually every aspect of life and adds greatly to the understanding of things we encounter. It therefore seems likely that we acquire knowledge both through direct experience and through secondary cognitive reflection in which additional relationships may be discovered.

As indicated, short-term memory enables thoughts arriving in consciousness at slightly different times to be held for comparison with each other. This enables common associations to be identified, thus establishing previously unrecognized relationships. The ability of short-term memory to function as a reservoir for ideas entering consciousness could provide another important function for the brain. Several thoughts arriving over a period of seconds to minutes could be retained and mixed within this modality. Whole or partial recombined memories could be sent into the unconscious processing area for a mixed interpretation. Their evaluation would be accomplished, as for any sensory perception. Any meaning derived would be based upon the new combination of memories generated in consciousness. In essence, short-term memory would enable the brief retention of separate thoughts, so they could be mixed for combined evaluation. This would seem to be an important part of normal thinking. Multiple thoughts arriving from the unconscious could be processed continuously in this way, yielding new combinations of ideas on each cycle. Long trains of thought would be perpetuated in this manner. In essence, the process of thinking may involve a constant recombining and mixing of ideas in consciousness, leading to new interpretations, and so forth.

CONSCIOUS AND UNCONSCIOUS PHASES OF THOUGHT

Thinking has been characterized here as a cyclic process involving both conscious and unconscious phases. In the previous paragraph, the mixing of memories in consciousness to generate new thoughts was discussed. This is probably a central process to normal thinking. Once memories are recombined, they are routed back to the unconscious interpretative areas for further processing. It is here that the matching and localization process occurs, yielding an interpretation for the new, blended memory. Information generated in this way would enter consciousness, where it could be recombined with even more memories to repeat the cycle, if desired. In essence, normal thinking appears to be generated from both conscious and unconscious forms of information processing. These will be more completely characterized in the following paragraphs.

The mechanism by which information is manipulated in consciousness has been described. Through this process, virtually any memory entering consciousness can be mixed with any other to yield a new interpretation. Because of the nature of the proposed process, there would be no necessity for memories combined in this way to have any prior association with each other. Totally unrelated memories could be called into consciousness to participate in this mixing process. In contrast, the information processing that occurs in the unconscious phase would have different restrictions. Data from consciousness, entering the interpretative areas, would initially be subject to localization and matching. Overlapped structures would undergo activation, triggering only associated structures. Unlike the mechanism proposed for consciousness, this phase of information processing would utilize only those memories linked in association. Unassociated memories would not be spontaneously activated unless they had previously been combined in consciousness. The flow of neural energy would thus follow lines of association, permitting only related memories to be involved in this form of processing.

It has been proposed that two types of data processing are utilized by the brain during normal thinking. In the conscious phase, whole or partial memories can be combined to produce new thoughts. There would be no requirement for such component memories to have any associated relationship prior to their mixing. Totally unconnected memories could be called into consciousness and compared or recombined in a variety of ways. In the unconscious phase, there would be no spontaneous mixing. Thoughts would be processed exactly as they came from consciousness. Interpretations of such thoughts would occur as associated memories of overlapped structures were activated. In this phase, associated organization would determine which memories were activated and entered consciousness as a subsequent thought. These two phases of information processing would operate in unison to produce thought and memory storage. This concept may be enormously important to mental function, as will be discussed.

A HYPOTHETICAL ORGANISM

Associated memories, which are utilized in the unconscious phase of information processing, provide a reference to prior experience. They maintain a record of the events that occur in our lives. Every new event or thought we experience is interpreted via this storehouse of data. All conclusions derived from this source are based closely upon what has transpired before. To better understand this concept, let us imagine a *hypothetical organism,* capable of using only this form of data manipulation. Conscious information processing, as postulated to exist in humans, would not be available, or would, perhaps, be of very poor quality. In such a situation, memories of past events could be stored and referenced with no difficulty. New events resembling those stored in memory could be adequately interpreted. This would provide the animal with sufficient data to evaluate and react appropriately to common situations. Such an organism would, however, be limited in other ways. Without the ability to compare memories in consciousness, subtle relationships could not be realized. Understanding of the world would be restricted largely to those things that were obvious at the time they occurred and entered memory. Mental concepts would therefore be very concrete, because only gross relationships could be appreciated. Because the ability to consciously process information would be poorly developed, subtle relationships would rarely be recognized. Such an organism's understanding of the world would be very superficial and consist largely of those things learned directly through experience. This, of course, would be a consequence of its inability to use the conscious type of information processing described here.

An organism like this would not be able to think in the conventional way. It would be able to activate memories, if triggered by an appropriate stimulus, but it would be unable to recombine these to produce new thoughts. In effect, its orientation would be very much limited to the here and now. Sensory perceptions would trigger memories that would provide interpretations applicable to the present. Its mental orientation would be primarily reactive. Concepts requiring cognitive analysis would not be possible, because conscious processing would be so poorly developed. There could be no appreciation for such things that could not be seen, touched, or directly sensed in some way. As such, there would be no awareness of such abstractions as self, mortality, time, and numerous others. These, of course, are ideas born largely through cognitive insight rather than direct experience. An appreciation of these concepts would therefore be impossible. Such an organism could not fantasize or plan for the future, because these skills require the conscious combination of memories. Existence for such creatures would be centered on the present. It is doubtful that there would be any real awareness of the passage of time. Cognitive skills would be necessary to integrate the past with the present, and to predict those events that might occur in the future. Organisms such as this would be very primitive by human standards. Despite these limitations, many forms of animal life on the earth today probably employ this form of mental organization.

THE ORIGIN OF TRUE THINKING

True thinking probably arose when the ability to recombine memories produced during unconscious processing evolved. The same evolutionary developments enabled memories retained in consciousness to be compared and subtle relationships to be realized. In essence, a second form of data processing was added to the original primitive system, allowing a vast expansion of mental capacity. Through these changes, it became possible to learn through cognitive reflection as well as direct experience. Language, representing a combination of ideas expressed verbally, became possible. Through the combination and comparison of ideas held in consciousness, associations between memories unrelated in direct experience became possible. It was no longer necessary for two events to occur within close temporal proximity for shared relationships to be realized. This form of analysis provided great insight. The brain became capable of seeing itself in a grander prospective. The concepts of self, mortality, death, and time were born. An awareness developed of the world that was not possible with the original form of data manipulation. Through the combination of these two forms of information processing, man became truly conscious.

RECOMBINATION OF MEMORIES
TO PRODUCE THOUGHT

According to this hypothesis, the mixing of unassociated memories would not occur in the unconscious memory-storage regions. Only those thoughts submitted to consciousness could be recombined to produce thinking. In this manner, both conscious and unconscious regions of the brain would be involved in the flow of thought. Thinking is much more than the mere recall of memories. Any tape recorder or computer can do this. As discussed, unconscious information processing may function in this way. Thinking, as we know it, seems to involve the recombination of these memories to yield new meaning and is probably only possible by combining conscious and unconscious systems. We utilize this type of mental activity when fantasies are created, or during the formulation of plans for the future. It is also a key component in problem solving. Various solutions can be proposed by recombining memories to generate different scenarios that fit any given situation. Each new arrangement of events can be assessed for feasibility and correctness through the interpretation process. This can be repeated numerous times, until an adequate solution is discovered. This is obviously an important and frequently used part of normal thought.

UNCONSCIOUS INFORMATION PROCESSING IN MAN

In the previous discussion, unconscious information processing is characterized as a somewhat mechanical reaction to thoughts formulated in consciousness. All responses result from the overlapping of corresponding structures, producing the activation of associated memories. There would be no freedom to combine unrelated memories in this realm. This would strictly be a function of consciousness. In most animals, thinking would be relatively simple. Their storehouses of information would be derived largely through direct experience rather than cognitive processing. In man, the situation would be quite different. New memories and relationships established through the combination of thoughts in consciousness would become part of this unconscious warehouse of knowledge. In other words, both cognitive conclusions originating in consciousness and factual material arising from direct experience would be available for reference through memory storage. Because of this, unconscious processing in man would be anything but unsophisticated. Interpretations based on memories arising from cognitive reflection would now be possible at an unconscious level. The process would still utilize associated memories, but the relationships of these entities to each other would be much more complex than in organisms with less well-developed conscious processing. In essence, conscious manipulation of data would serve to *program* this unconscious storehouse of memories, making a sophisticated level of interpretation possible.

CYCLIC GENERATION OF LANGUAGE

The principles described may also play a role in language formulation and its expression in speech or thought. Sentences might be constructed in consciousness by linking successive words or groups of words as they cycle from the unconscious interpretation area. The following sequence of events can be postulated. Words or short phrases would enter consciousness, where they would be briefly stored in short-term memory. Here they would be sequentially combined with other words, arriving from the interpretation areas, to form sentences. Each cycle of thought would add one or more words, so that complete sentences would be built, piece by piece. Cycling would be rapid, and the process would be perceived by the thinker as continuous and uninterrupted. After the addition of each new word or phrase, the entire assembly would again undergo interpretation, which would stimulate the release of more words. These would travel back into consciousness and be linked to the stem words that produced their release. This new grouping would again undergo interpretation, stimulating more words to be produced, and the process would continue. Each cycle of thought would lengthen the sentence somewhat. Each new addition of words would be followed by an interpretation phase, and so on. Every turn of the cycle would add one or more words, allowing full sentences to be constructed in consciousness. As described before, short-term memory would be an important part of this process. It would enable words to be held in place during the construction of sentences. Without it, only short phrases would seem possible. Long sentences would be partially forgotten by the time they were completed.

Along these same lines, Baddeley proposed a model for working memory (short-term memory) in 1986 that included an auditory subsystem specialized for speech. He referred to this component of working memory as the *articulatory loop*. This system facilitates the processing of sentences by holding words so that larger chunks of information can be added, and the material can be rehearsed prior to its verbal expression. Baddeley felt each articulatory loop had a duration of no more than about 2 seconds, during which time words held in a temporary store were rehearsed in loop fashion. He postulated that this system could function subvocally as the inner voice we recognize during verbal thought.

As indicated earlier, language seems to represent a shorthand way of expressing nonverbal memories and thoughts. It probably originated solely to facilitate communication between people. Whenever language is used, the brain is attempting to describe its basic sensory memories in a way that can be readily understood by others. This is the driving force behind the formation of sentences, as just described. The words that leave the interpretation areas and enter consciousness are translations of nonverbal thought. The brain is attempting to describe in words the things it inwardly sees. On each cycle this verbal description would be stored in short-term memory. When it reenters the interpretation areas, it would again be converted back into nonverbal terms and checked for accuracy with the original reference. This would stimulate additional verbal description, which would again cycle into consciousness, as described. This process would, of course, involve both conscious and unconscious forms of information processing, as discussed before.

The hypothesis presented suggests that language serves as an interface between the external world and the inner brain. Words sensed through the ears are unconsciously converted into their basic meanings, so that the information conveyed can be processed. Once this is completed, a reverse translation process occurs, and the information derived is converted back into word form for outward expression. This process seems complex, but is based upon the idea that nonverbal information processing preceded the development of language. The expression of ideas in words simply represents a refinement to the preexisting system. This seems analogous to one aspect of computer organization. Commands expressed in human language are entered into these devices and converted into digital codes, which can be utilized by the circuits of the computer. Information is processed in this analog form and converted back into words for our convenience. In this type of system, language also seems to function as an interface linking two separate functional domains.

LANGUAGE MAY ARISE FROM ASSOCIATED MEMORIES

In keeping with the proposed hypothesis, we can speculate that each word in language is probably associated in memory with other words to which it is linked through usage. Some words are frequently grouped together and would be strongly associated. Others are weakly associated, whereas a few may never be paired in usage and show no association. In essence, each word expressed as a GMC will be linked in memory with a number of other words that show varying degrees of association. Each successive word of a sentence may be chosen from this associated list of words. The last word of a partial sentence being cycled through the interpretation area may determine the next word to be added from its associated list. The one chosen may best describe the nonverbal thought being translated. It is likely that this would be the word with the highest degree of association that adequately describes the situation. In this way, sentences may be constructed by the movement of thought down lines of association, as described for other mental processes. The last word of each partial sentence would trigger its matching GMC, which, in turn, would activate its associations. From these associated words, the one most descriptive of the nonverbal idea is somehow chosen and released into consciousness. Perhaps this would be the word most strongly associated with the nonverbal idea being described. This would allow the choice of a word to depend both on the strength of association with the previous word and the nonverbal reference. This would seem to be the most suitable arrangement. In some cases, several closely associated words may be grouped in a single GMC, and released as a unit, adding several words to the growing sentence.

The process, described for the construction of sentences, involves the successive linking of associated elements. This may be the exact process that guides the synthesis of fantasies, as indicated in an earlier chapter. Each unit of a fantasy, or word of a sentence, is chosen from a list of items held in association with the preceding word, or memory. This list contains all options previously acquired through experience. In a fantasy, each successive piece may be chosen by the emotion evoked or the desirability of the final outcome of the events as arranged. Fantasies are probably constructed in a cyclic manner, as proposed for the construction of sentences. Like sentences, fantasies can be altered at will if the interpretation phase of each cycle indicates that the ideas being expressed are not exactly as desired. This provides the flexibility we are familiar with in thought. It should be noted that the ability of the brain to recombine visual or verbal elements to generate new fantasies, or sentences, is probably mediated through the property of *generativity*, which was described earlier in this chapter.

MECHANISMS OF THOUGHT

A number of mechanisms for the movement of thought have been proposed in this chapter, each with a slightly different purpose. In reality, these mechanisms probably do not exist separately. Thought is probably a blend of each in various proportions. In reality, they probably do not exist in pure form, as described, but are integrated to produce coherent thought. There is probably extensive overlap in these processes. In support of this concept is the idea that all mechanisms proposed here operate in the same basic way. There is an initial localization and matching process, followed by an interpretation phase and transport of any new conclusions to consciousness and short-term memory. This process can repeat itself with slight variations to accomplish the functions of thought presented in this hypothesis.

It seems possible that the process by which memory fragments are recombined in consciousness to form new thoughts may be directed by a *feedback-type mechanism.* Perhaps a number of memories have been reviewed in consciousness that bear on some question that requires a response. Fragments of these memories, held in short-term memory, may be combined to produce new thoughts in an attempt to better understand the situation. On each cycle of thought, the resulting interpretation may guide the composition of subsequent combinations. In effect, the process may be one of successive approximation. Each round of thought would progressively refine the existing combination of memories until an adequate interpretation was found. In essence, the process may be one of continuous feedback and revision. As most of us are aware, problem solving is frequently a process of trial and error which continues until an adequate solution is found.

OVERVIEW OF CONCEPTS

In an effort to create a conceptualized basis for thought, many separate ideas have been proposed here and in earlier chapters. Perhaps these entities might be better understood in relationship to each other by a brief overview of the concepts presented so far. In this work, thoughts are viewed as various combinations of memories created by the flow of ideas through consciousness. As thinking occurs, the memories and partial memories that compose such thoughts accumulate in short-term memory. This would allow entities arriving in consciousness at different times to mix and form new combinations. Short-term memory would make this possible. These new arrangements would then be electrically transmitted to the unconscious interpretive areas, where localization and matching with stored memories would occur. These areas might be visualized as vast seas of overlapping neural patterns, representing our stores of accumulated memories. This is consistent with the idea that memories are groupings of associations that are more electrically conductive with each other than with surrounding associations and are stored in overlapping fashion with similar structures.

The smallest units of memory present in these areas would be extensively utilized as structural elements in memory. Each might serve as a functional part of literally thousands of larger, individual structures of many sizes. Such small units would be linked with other structures to form progressively larger memories. The complexities and sizes of memories would, of course, be dictated by experience. We can imagine that there would be extensive partial and whole overlapping of structures as similar memories were laid down on top of each other through years of experience.

As indicated in an earlier chapter, matching would initially begin with the smallest pieces of data present in the new thought. Piece by piece, small corresponding structures (GMCs) would be matched and overlapped in memory storage. Each small unit activated in this way would send energy to its many associations. Many larger structures would receive some stimulation in this way. Larger structures that received sufficient stimulation would be activated. Of course, many smaller structures might be necessary to produce total activation of such structures. Once activated, associations specific only for these larger structures as intact whole units would receive transmitted energy. These would then combine with other activated associations to provide stimulation for even larger units of memory. This would continue until all possible structures were matched. The final result would, of course, be a function of how closely the original information from consciousness corresponded to past experience, as recorded in memory. Such identified structures would then enter consciousness and serve as the interpretation for the original thought. According to this mechanism, structures of progressively greater size would be stimulated, until a maximum fit of the original data from consciousness was achieved. The process would strive to activate the largest memories possible to ensure a maximum level of understanding. Such an interpretation might then recombine with memories still in short-term memory, or be mixed with new thoughts and undergo another round of interpretation. This cyclic process could be repeated numerous times. Each new combination of memories would provide a new interpretation that, in turn, might further perpetuate the process.

It has been proposed in this chapter that information processing in the human brain involves both conscious and unconscious neural activity. A model has been presented in which information moves in a sequential and integrated manner from one realm to the next to achieve the goals of thought. In the hypothetical animal brain that was described, human information processing and consciousness would not exist. Sensory perceptions that entered the brain would be matched to existing memories to produce interpretations and any necessary actions. Such a system would enable these organisms to learn through experience and adequately deal with routine environmental conditions, even though there would be no active awareness of these processes. Many primitive organisms probably exist today that employ this type of mental organization in some form.

Despite such an organism's ability to cope and survive, it would be incapable of *true* human consciousness and thought. Its mental activity world be largely restricted to the *immediate present,* and behavior would be *reactive* in nature. In such a system, cyclic thought would not be possible because of the absence of the *feedback circuitry* postulated to exist in the human brain. Sensory perceptions would result in interpretations and any necessary behavioral responses. The sequence of neural activity would end at this point and would only resume when challenged by a new perception. In contrast, human interpretations arising from incoming data would feed back through the appropriate sensory perception areas, where they would be reprocessed in the same way as new perceptions. In effect, interpretations would undergo reinterpretation as single entities or in combination with other associations held in short-term memory to produce conscious thoughts with new meanings. This recombination process was previously discussed.

AWARENESS AS A FUNCTION OF FEEDBACK CIRCUITRY

Through this cyclic arrangement, the brain would see its interpretations and be aware of its own conclusions. *Awareness* would be a consequence of this form of closed circuitry. In this way, the brain would *know that it knew.* Long chains of cyclic thought, related through association, would sequentially arise through unconscious processing and enter awareness via reinterpretation. By folding neural activity back upon itself in this way, information processing would not stop after each interpretation, as in the primitive organism, but might continue, until all aspects of the original perception were considered. Past situations and considerations might be mixed with current perceptions to provide a wider range of behavioral options, which should also be subject to greater volitional control. Through this process, life events would become temporally integrated to produce the awareness and mental flexibility that is characteristic of conscious experience.

In the model presented, consciousness is assumed to occupy no centralized location within the brain. In other words, no mysterious higher command center or executive brain region, as depicted by some older models, is proposed. Conscious perception is felt to be a natural byproduct of the interpretative process to which all information passing through the brain is exposed. In effect, consciousness is considered to be an ongoing, dynamic process that arises when interpretations are cycled back through the brain via feedback circuitry. Through this process, it is reasonable that the brain may develop an awareness of its own inner workings and cognitive conclusions. This scenario suggests that consciousness itself may essentially be an *interpretation.* The feedback circuitry described here may be anatomically similar to the *reentry pathways* proposed by Gerald Edelman in *The Remembered Present: A Biological Theory of Consciousness* (1989).

BLINDSIGHT

The phenomenon of *blindsight* may help to understand the concepts presented here. For many years, it has been recognized that destruction of the primary visual area (striate cortex), located in the occipital lobes of the cerebral cortex, produces blindness, even though the eyes and optic nerves may remain intact. Individuals afflicted with such *cortical blindness* completely deny any conscious perception of visual stimuli. In addition, they act and appear totally sightless under normal circumstances. Despite this, such individuals can successfully perform certain visual tasks, even though they continue to insist that they see nothing. Often they can distinguish between vertical, horizontal, and diagonal lines, as well as simple forms, colors, and relative positions of objects, with a high degree of accuracy. In such cases, there is an obvious dissociation between the conscious perception of vision and the ability to perform tasks requiring sight.

In humans, as well as monkeys, several visual pathways have been identified that lead from the optic nerves to various parts of the cortex. When the primary visual cortex is destroyed, it is generally assumed that secondary visual areas residing within the cortex may still receive some visual stimulation via these alternate or supplemental routes. In this way, some information from the eyes may still enter the brain, allowing some visual tasks to be performed by those with cortical blindness. Although conscious awareness of such information is absent, its presence within the brain can be demonstrated by testing.

Although this explanation for blindsight is commonly accepted, it is obviously incomplete, in that it provides little insight into the apparent loss of visual consciousness. As postulated earlier in this work, the primary visual area (sensory perception area for vision), located in the posterior occipital lobes, may constitute a portion of the feedback circuit allowing visual memories to gain access to consciousness. Destruction of this cortical structure should short-circuit the feedback of information necessary to establish awareness. Such a damaged visual system should functionally resemble that of the hypothetical organism described previously. In other words, conscious awareness of a visual perception would not be generated, even though the information itself would be registered in memory storage. In effect, incoming visual data would undergo matching and localization with memories in storage, but the resulting interpretation would be unable to cycle through the brain to produce conscious awareness. Such an arrangement is consistent with other ideas presented in this work and seems to provide a rational explanation for the loss of visual consciousness in blindsight. The participation of the visual cortex in conscious experience is also consistent with the ideas of G. William Farthing. In his 1992 book entitled *The Psychology of Consciousness,* he states, in reference to blindsight, that "the implication is that only the primary visual pathway, via the striate cortex, connects to brain circuits that generate conscious visual experience" (p. 132). In Figure 4.4, the flow of data within the brain as it may occur in blindsight is illustrated.

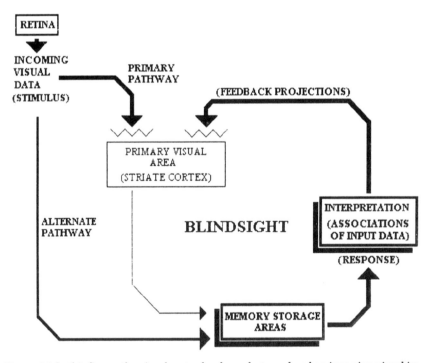

Figure 4.4 In this figure, the visual cortex has been destroyed and an incoming visual image travels via an alternate pathway to memory storage. Localization occurs, and an interpretation is produced in a normal way. In the absence of the visual cortex, the normal cyclic path (see Figure 4.1) is disrupted and the interpretation never reaches consciousness. Presumably, this interpretation is still available at some level within the brain, producing the phenomenon of blindsight.

BLIND-TOUCH

It also seems probable that memories of smell, touch, hearing, and those originating from other sensory modalities may also enter primary consciousness in much the same way as do visual memories. In other words, feedback of nonvisual memories through their appropriate sensory perception areas may be a necessary requirement for such entities to gain conscious awareness. This is supported by the fact that *blind-touch*, which is the tactile equivalent of blindsight, has been observed (Paillard, Michel, & Stelmach, 1983).

CONCLUDING REMARKS

A number of principles have been proposed in this chapter to explain the generation and flow of thought within the brain and the development of primary consciousness. The processes involved appear complex but are certainly not unreasonable, based on our current knowledge of neuroscience. The essence of thinking appears to employ a cyclic framework, utilizing both conscious and unconscious regions of the brain. Thoughts or sensory perceptions held in consciousness can be sent into the unconscious interpretative areas, where similar memories can be localized and used to provide interpretation. Meaning can come from single memories or be derived from many in combination. This provides the flexibility necessary to deal with the intricacies of daily life in the many situations we encounter. All interpretations of current issues are based on prior experience, as stored in memory. By transferring this stored knowledge from similar past situations to the present, understanding is achieved in terms already familiar to the brain. Thoughts and sensory data held in short-term memory can be recombined to provide mixed interpretations unique to their combination. This process seems to be the source of new ideas characteristic of human thought. In addition, previously unidentified relationships can also be determined by the identification of common associations held by larger ideas. This is probably the basis for abstract and creative thinking.

In this work, conscious awareness is viewed as a by-product of the evaluation process to which all information passing through the brain is subjected. The feedback of unconscious interpretations through the various sensory perception areas may be essential to the development of primary consciousness by allowing such data to become visible to the brain. In combination, the mechanisms described in this chapter seem to adequately capture the essence of conscious experience and the dynamic processes that govern associative thinking.

Emotions

Emotions function as mental sensations that add richness and emphasis to the many things we experience. Through their expression, life is truly felt and understood at a basic, nonspoken level. In this chapter, a theory of emotion will be presented that is consistent with this concept as well as the *association hypothesis*. Emotions will be characterized as *associations of memories* that provide them with a basic level of *interpretation*. It will be further suggested that emotions collectively constitute an *inner language* that motivates thought and allows us to appreciate and interpret the many events we continuously experience. In effect, they will be characterized as a *nonverbal form of mental communication* that preceded and eventually led to the development of spoken language.

BACKGROUND

Perhaps the first modern consideration of this subject came from Charles Darwin (1872/1965) in *The Expression of the Emotions in Man and Animals*, in which he attempted to trace the origins of emotional responses as they were related to facial expression. The first formal theory of emotion was proposed by William James (an American psychologist) and Carl Lange (a Danish physiologist) working independently. The James–Lange theory suggests that emotion is the mental perception of somatic and visceral changes occurring in the body (James, 1884, 1890). For example, sorrow is generated by crying, fear results from trembling, and so forth. In contrast to what seems intuitive, this theory suggests that life events produce somatic changes, which, in turn, result in the perception of emotion. This theory received recent support in a book entitled *Emotions: A Reconsideration of Somatic Theory* (1989) by A.C. Papanicolaou. Other theories have suggested that changes in facial expression can produce corresponding emotional responses (Izard, 1977, 1981, 1982; Leventhal, 1982).

The Cannon–Bard theory of emotion evolved largely because of dissatisfaction with the James–Lange hypothesis. It was originally proposed by Walter B. Cannon in 1929 and extended by Bard in 1938. The hypothesis suggests that events activate the thalamus, which, in turn, sends signals to the body and cerebral cortex. As a result, emotional arousal and somatic stimulation occur simultaneously rather than in sequence, as proposed by James and Lange. In a later work by Plutchik (1980), it was suggested that the hypothalamus and limbic system, rather than the thalamus, may be central to emotional expression. In addition, Plutchik proposed that eight essential emotions exist in humans, which can be combined in various proportions to produce all the others.

Through the years, other theories of emotion have been proposed (Angyal, 1941; DeRivera, 1977; Frijda, 1986; Schachter & Singer, 1962; Scherer, 1988; Smith & Ellsworth, 1985; Weiner, 1985). One such hypothesis is the *affect theory*, originally proposed by Tomkins in 1962 and 1963. Using this theory, recent attempts have been made to explain the emotional disruptions seen in some forms of psychiatric illness (Stone, 1993) and to understand the role of emotion in cognitive (Milestone, 1993) as well as drug therapy (Nathanson & Pfrommer, 1993). (For a general overview of affect theory, see Nathanson, 1993.) Despite this work, there is still a great deal of confusion and uncertainty about this fascinating aspect of mental activity. The theory of emotion presented here is based on the associated nature of mental entities, as proposed in earlier chapters.

DIFFERENTIAL EMOTIONS THEORY

Perhaps the hypothesis with the most current relevance in neuroscience today is C. E. Izard's *differential emotions theory* (1971,1977). Izard effectively integrates a wide range of concepts and observations into a compelling theoretical framework of emotion. Some of the important similarities between Izard's theory and the ideas that will be presented here can be summarized as follows:

1. Emotions function as motivators of action and behavior. In this role they promote survival and well-being by working in combi-

nation with such natural drives as hunger, pain avoidance, and sexual desire.

2. There are a limited number of fundamental or innate emotions. In differential emotion theory, 10 such emotions are identified. These include interest/excitement, joy, surprise, sadness, anger, disgust, contempt, fear, shame, and guilt.

3. Fundamental emotions can combine to produce cumulative mental effects. For example, differential emotions theory defines anxiety as fear combined with two or more emotions, such as anger, sadness, guilt or shame, and the positive emotion of interest/excitement. In a like manner, depression is considered to be a combination of sadness, anger, disgust, contempt, fear, shyness, and guilt.

4. Emotions, like reflexes, instincts, and drives, have evolved because they provide a selective survival advantage through their ability to motivate and protect

5. Emotions provide drive and direction for thought, which can be expressed in behavior.

6. Emotions or feelings can exist in association with memories. In differential emotions theory, such complexes are termed affective–cognitive structures.

7. Emotions are considered to have a genetic origin. In differential emotions theory, this assumption is based on the observation that emotional expression in widely diverse cultures, even those that are isolated and preliterate, is essentially the same. This, of course, suggests that emotion has a common neural basis that transcends cultural lines.

In subsequent pages, an attempt will be made to integrate these concepts into the association theory that is proposed here. In addition, new ideas will be introduced, which I hope will provide an expanded framework for the study of this complex subject.

OVERVIEW OF EMOTIONS

In this work, emotions are considered to serve several purposes. Through their ability to motivate, they stimulate cognitive mental activity. In essence, emotions are viewed here as the main drivers of thought. They also function as mental markers, which tell us the importance previously associated with any given memory. In this way, they provide a form of interpretation for similar current situations. These functions will be discussed in detail. Their last purpose is to stimulate autonomic responses in the organism through the peripheral release of various catecholamines. This, of course, is a well-established biological principle, which is critical to survival. In this work, the primary focus will be on emotion generated during thought and the intake of sensory data. Noncognitive routes to emotional activation will also be briefly considered.

In this chapter, the relationship of thought and emotion will be explored. It seems likely that neither entity can have full meaning without the other. Thought and emotion probably coexist in an *interwoven relationship*, which permits normal cognitive functioning. This interdependency has long been suspected by many psychiatrists and others who study human thought. Their blending in the brain determines what we think and our subsequent actions. In a sense, emotions direct our lives by allowing us to distinguish important from trivial matters. They convey appropriateness and relevance to our thinking, allowing us to assess current situations and make the numerous value judgments necessary to cope with life. In effect, normal thinking is guided by our emotional interpretations. By examining pathological states in which emotion is disrupted, this important relationship can be easily observed. This will be attempted in the next few pages. Much can also be learned by observing normal thought. The evidence suggests that emotion is far from being a dying remnant of the past. It is a central driver of thought and action, and is basic to our very existence and survival.

EMOTION IN POSTTRAUMATIC STRESS DISORDER

Perhaps we should first examine some of the ways emotions, thoughts, and memories are known to be related. It is generally realized that the durability of a new memory is directly related to the intensity and quality of the emotion experienced at the time of storage. Events that evoke strong emotion produce memories that often endure a lifetime, without the necessity for repetition or rehearsal. This type of memory storage is obvious in pathological states such as posttraumatic stress disorder (PTSD). By definition, the events that produce this condition are so extreme as to be classified outside the range of normal human experience (American Psychiatric Association, 1987). They are often related to wartime trauma or childhood sexual abuse. Such memories are often experienced as painful flashbacks, which may recur for many years after the original events. These memories are often so durable and emotionally charged that they cannot be adequately repressed or dealt with effectively by the brain's normal defense mechanisms. Unfortunately, this disorder is not uncommon, and it is very difficult to treat effectively.

PTSD illustrates an extreme example of the brain's ability to retain memories of events stored under intense emotion. This relationship between emotional intensity and memory storage is, however, probably not pathological, under most circumstances. It appears to represent a normal mental process that is important to the routine storage of information. From general observation, the intensity of emotion evoked by events in life seems to determine the ultimate strength of the resulting memory. Without this property, our memory stores would lack information about the significance of past events. In effect, all memories would be stored with equal strength. Trivial events would be no more retrievable than those essential for survival, and important memories would have no more durability than those of less significance. By pairing emotional intensity with memory storage, information can be retained in a way that gives priority to important things. It is therefore suggested that the intensity of emotion may serve to mark a memory's significance. This would appear important to survival. Without this mental process, the meaningful things in life would have no more obvious value and produce no more durable memories than the enormous volume of routine and trivial events we encounter daily. In a sense, each memory we store is probably classified by its associated emotion. The nature of an emotion associated with a memory provides an interpretation of past events, and the intensity tells us about its prior importance. The pairing of memories with emotion would seem to have obvious biological value.

EMOTION IN DEPRESSION

Major depression is an illness that affects the expression and quality of emotion, and is generally felt to represent a primary disturbance of mood (the dominant, subjective emotional tone experienced over time) rather than thought. In the more severe forms of this illness, patients experience a total lack of pleasure. Their dominant emotional tone is negative. They often feel unremitting despair, frustration, and sadness. Their inability to control these feelings often produces a profound sense of helplessness and hopelessness. There is usually a total absence of normal happiness or joy, even for brief periods. Although depression is generally considered to be an illness of mood, in severe cases, the content of thought may also be affected. The patient will often dwell on painful memories of the past. The small, normal irritations of life may seem monumental. Insignificant tasks often become overwhelming. Small slights from others take on unrealistic proportions. Common things, which are normally dealt with easily, may become interpreted as major events that can not be readily surmounted. In effect, normal thinking and judgment can also be altered as a consequence of this illness. There are often major changes in the patient's mood as well as thinking.

As the illness progresses, additional changes in thought can occur. Patients may become obsessed with ideas of death and even suicide. Their judgment and insight often become severely impaired. Their entire view of the world may become shaped by the unrelenting emotional pain they experience. Thought, and even physical movement, may become visibly and subjectively slowed. Thinking may become laborious, and thoughts frequently are lost from the brain before they can be completely expressed. Memory may deteriorate as concentration becomes more difficult. Eventually the patient may lose touch with reality. Symptoms of *psychosis*, such as auditory hallucinations and delusions, often develop. Some patients may experience irrational fears of family or friends. Paranoia or unrealistic guilt may ensue. Some patients become catatonic and require extensive nursing care to prevent death. It is obvious that thought and emotion are both closely interwoven in this illness. As emotion deteriorates, thought content changes, and eventually a psychosis may develop. At this point, a major deterioration in the patient's mental status will be evident. Treatment usually requires hospitalization.

EMOTION IN MANIA

A different relationship seems to exist between thought and emotion in patients in the *manic phase* of bipolar mood disorder. In contrast to depression, thoughts seem to race through the brain, often jumping from one subject to the next. Mental activity can be so rapid that patients often will comment that they are unable to talk fast enough to keep up with their thoughts. Their speech is often so rapid and jumbled that it is incoherent. As indicated before, in depression, thoughts are perceived as sluggish and laborious. Speech may be very slow and tedious. This is in direct contrast to the manic patient. The types of emotion experienced in each state may also be completely opposite. Manic patients are frequently on top of the world, although anger and other energizing negative emotions may also be present. They often feel invincible and able to overcome any obstacle. Their energy often seems boundless, and they may require only a few hours of sleep a night. Everything seems speeded up and magnified in their lives. Their thoughts may be grandiose, and they may see their normal abilities in a greatly exaggerated way. Often they unrealistically feel that anything can be accomplished. As in depression, there is a distortion in thought that parallels changes in mood.

Patients experiencing mania may also progress to frank psychosis. They often display the same gross disruptions of reality seen in depression. These observations have led many people to feel that depression and mania may be opposite ends of the same spectrum. In one case, thought and speech become dramatically slowed as the brain becomes preoccupied with dysphoric emotion. In the opposite situation, thought and speech are greatly accelerated as the dominate emotional tone becomes more positive or energized. In both cases, these distortions in thought often lead to a failure to distinguish real from unreal, and psychosis ensues.

In these illnesses there is obviously a strong link between thought and emotion. One cannot vary without an alteration in the other. This interdependency supports the idea that emotion is not simply a way of driving autonomic responses in the periphery of the body. Emotions are an integral part of what we know as thought. They function together, allowing us to understand the world in which we live. Thoughts without emotional interpretations are as sterile as the printout from a computer. Words convey a certain amount of information, but their full understanding and significance is not possible without an emotional component. It seems possible that the distortions in thought observed in depression and mania may be the result of emotional interpretations that are faulty. As a consequence, the content of further thought is altered, and frank misinterpretations of reality eventually become apparent.

EMOTION IN SCHIZOPHRENIA

Schizophrenia is a devastating type of psychiatric illness, which is characterized by a chronic psychosis. In contrast to depression, the underlying defect is felt to involve a primary disturbance in thought form rather than emotion. Although this illness can exist in several related variations, patients will frequently experience auditory or visual hallucinations, delusions, paranoia, and various bizarre forms of behavior. The common thread that links all forms of schizophrenia is the failure to appreciate and distinguish reality. Patients may experience auditory hallucinations, which may be misinterpreted as voices of the dead, or have elaborate delusional systems made up of false beliefs integrated into other nonpsychotic aspects of life. There is often much confusion, because they are unable to distinguish dreams or inner thoughts from externally occurring events. In some way, they are unable to maintain a normal internal representation of the world for reference.

Despite the gross distortion of thought that characterizes this illness, there is often an easily detectable disturbance of emotion. This observation has been described in the literature for many years and is well documented. Patients with certain forms of this illness display a greatly reduced level of emotional energy, as indicated by a flat, unchanging affect. Facial expressions generally show little variation during conversation, and speech is often flat and monotonic. There is a complete absence of normal emotional expression in many cases. Because this important aspect of normal communication is lacking, these patients are often difficult to understand. In addition to an overall reduction in emotional tone, the emotion that remains is often inappropriate. A patient may laugh when talking about some tragic event, or cry when describing a normally joyful situation. There is an obvious mismatch between emotion and thought in many cases.

Schizophrenia provides another example of the interwoven nature of thought and emotion. When one deteriorates as the result of a disease process, the other also shows some degree of distortion. The two do not appear to exist separately. From these observations, it is not possible to determine their exact relationship, but it is obvious that in some way they are interdependent. It seems unlikely that one can be altered without some change in the other. Once again, this suggests that thinking is probably dependent on both factors for normal expression.

EMOTION IN OBSESSIVE–COMPULSIVE DISORDER

Obsessive–compulsive disorder (OCD) is another psychiatric disorder that causes a considerable amount of distress (Rapoport, 1989). It is far from being uncommon, as once thought. Four million Americans are estimated to suffer from this illness at any one time. Its symptoms can range from mild to incapacitatingly severe. Patients with this illness experience recurrent, intrusive thoughts, accompanied by unrealistic fears and anxiety. These thoughts are so frequent as to be classified as obsessive. Patients literally cannot *let go*. They often ruminate constantly about seemingly insignificant details, which most people may consider once and put aside. The anxiety associated with this practice is often overwhelming and totally preoccupying. For obvious reasons, this is considered the obsessive portion of the disorder. In order to deal with the anxiety accompanying these thoughts, OCD patients may develop ritualistic activity. If they ruminate about closing the house up properly before leaving, a specific routine may emerge to ease their anxiety. They may develop a schedule for checking all the windows and doors in a certain sequence, which must be repeated several times before they are sure all is in order. Checking-type routines are frequent and may involve virtually any aspect of life. Some of these patients may have an exaggerated fear of bacterial or chemical contamination and may wash constantly to reduce the associated anxiety. OCD may take many forms, but it is generally characterized by obsessive thoughts accompanied by unrealistic fear and a type of compulsive behavior designed to partially alleviate this distress. Patients frequently see their behavior as silly but must continue it to reduce the level of anxiety. This appears to be a clear example of emotion acting as a driver for thought and subsequent behavior. The repetitive, intrusive thoughts continue to cycle through the brain because of the associated emotion that is released in this process. Patients fear a dreadful outcome if they do not pay adequate attention to the issues of concern.

Fortunately, new drug therapy has become available to help patients with OCD. Treatment with fluoxetine (Turner, Jacob, Beidel, & Himmelhoch, 1985) or clomipramine (Insel et al., 1983) dramatically reduces the symptoms in the majority of patients. It is felt that these drugs work by blocking the reuptake of serotonin in the synaptic connections between cells of the central nervous system. In effect, they alter brain chemistry by increasing the concentration of this neurotransmitter within synaptic clefts. In some way, this reduces the symptoms of OCD.

Much can be learned by talking with successfully treated OCD patients. They report that obsessive thoughts gradually fade over time when they take medication. They will often say that a thought may recur from time to time, but it no longer bothers them. The emotional component has either completely faded or has been greatly reduced. Because of this, the drive to repeat the thought and engage in compensatory behavior is lost. It is now simply a thought like any other. It no longer carries the emotional significance that perpetuated the original cycle. The driving force has been dissipated, providing great relief for the patient. In some way, these remarkable drugs seem to separate or uncouple the affective component of this illness from the thought. By observing this process, the significance of emotion coupled with thought can be directly viewed. Although OCD is an example of a pathological blending of these elements, most normal thoughts have associated emotion that define their meaning within the brain.

EMOTIONS AS MOTIVATORS OF THOUGHT
AND ACTION

Emotions are characterized here as the motivating force for all thought and action initiated in life. Perhaps this can be further illustrated by again considering schizophrenia. As indicated earlier, in this illness, there is generally a global reduction in the expression of emotion. These patients just do not seem capable of feeling things in a normal way. The emotion necessary for this seems largely absent. If emotion drives thought, these patients should show a diminished level of physical and mental activity. This is, in fact, exactly what can be observed in many cases. These patients generally show an ambivalence and lack of interest in normal activities. There is not a substitution by other activities but a generalized lack of interest in almost everything. Schizophrenia is frequently characterized as an *amotivational* state. Occasionally patients will be described as showing *poverty of thought*, indicating that there is little evidence of any cognitive activity. When challenged by an examiner, they frequently will be able to respond appropriately, indicating that this function is not totally lost. What seems to be absent is the ability to inwardly initiate or sustain a reasonable level of thought. Perhaps this is very difficult without a normal complement of emotion to drive the process. Of course, with an illness as complex as schizophrenia, it is difficult to determine any absolute cause and effect relationship. At this point, all we can say is that the symptoms described are well characterized and may be related as proposed.

In the past few pages, evidence has been presented suggesting that thought and emotion are closely related. Various pathological states have been examined, and a correlation seems obvious, at least in these cases. Evidence that emotion drives thought is particularly obvious in OCD. New, effective drug therapy for this disorder provides us with valuable insight into this relationship. In this illness, it actually seems possible to separate emotion from thought and observe the resulting changes. If we continue to examine this relationship in persons without major psychiatric pathology, this interdependency of emotion and thought also seems apparent. Let us look at some of the ways these entities are related in our everyday lives.

Is there any action or thought that is not at least indirectly driven by emotion? If we examine our activities and their motivations, the role of emotion becomes clearer. Ultimately everything we engage in seems guided by the unconscious drive to achieve a certain emotional state. Some obvious examples of this include music, movies, television, and books. We engage in these activities because of the emotional stimulation that results from our participation. Our hopes and dreams, the mates we choose, and the people we associate with, are largely selected to satisfy our emotional needs. We tailor our fantasies and choose our hobbies and life's work by how they make us feel. The heavy use of drugs and alcohol in our society can probability also be attributed to their ability to temporarily alter mood in a favorable way. This need to satisfy our emotional requirements is a basic, natural drive in all of us. It is so ingrained in our behavior that we are usually unaware of its continuous influence on the many choices we make. It is reflected in virtually every aspect of our lives. It could actually be argued that this is the basic drive that ultimately underlies all human behavior. It may be the single, most important motivator in life.

Although the biological nature of emotions is still largely obscure, these entities seem to be released into the brain in association with specific memories. In other words, the recall of memories frequently triggers certain emotions. This is a common occurrence and suggests that there is a biological and associative pairing of these elements within the brain. Such a system would allow each memory we possess to be linked with its emotional interpretation, as established at the time of memory storage. The sensory perception of an event would initiate the search and localization of a similar memory, as described before. It would be released into consciousness, along with any associated emotional component. The new event would therefore be interpreted as was the original reference memory. Once again, prior experience would be used to help understand the present. Without this accompanying emotional component, each memory would carry the same weight. We would have no more fear of a house cat than a wild tiger, although cognitively we might recognize the difference. In this way, emotion allows us to classify memories by relative importance. This has obvious survival advantage and is essential to everyday functioning. As indicated before, each memory's emotional component seems to determine its durability and prominence within the brain.

It seems likely that the emotion released when a memory is recalled serves to influence and direct further thought. A memory judged to be relevant to current issues may stimulate further thinking along the same lines. If the emotional component indicates that thoughts are of a trivial nature (i.e., not appropriate to the current situation), the direction of thinking may change. In a like manner, emotionally unpleasant thoughts may trigger a switch to more pleasant things. We may spend more time in creative, relaxing thinking than we do on unpleasant, anxiety-producing subjects. There are a multitude of subtle emotions that can guide thought in many different directions. Curiosity or interest may stimulate thinking, as may anxiety. Frustration may cause us to avoid a given subject or might stimulate thought in an effort to eliminate this feeling. Joy or pleasure might cause us to dwell on a certain memory or change our behavior in an effort to prolong or reproduce these emotions. Painful memories may be suppressed in an attempt to avoid the emotional component. Various mental tasks may be driven by the feeling of the satisfaction released. Plans may be initiated based upon the anticipation of certain desired emotions. We may even go to the dentist to avoid the unpleasant emotion associated with the pain of dental decay if we delay. The most likely conclusion that can be drawn from these and numerous similar examples is that thought and subsequent action is driven by emotion. Behavior, which is the ultimate manifestation of thought, is motivated by the emotion generated. It seems plausible that this simple premise is the ultimate driving force in our lives.

In today's technological world, emotions are somehow viewed as being out of step with modern life. They are often felt to be aging remnants of an older, more animalistic past. Today's man is somehow characterized as being beyond emotion. He is often portrayed in movies and television as a cold, detached being, who processes information much like a computer. In many situations, emotional expression is viewed as weak and something to be avoided, if possible. Most people who carefully examine these ideas realize how absurd they really are. Without emotions, we would be no more capable of independent thought and action than the average computer. Emotions color our experiences and allow interpretation not possible with sensory memories alone. They constitute the main quality of our intellect, which separates us from the artificial intelligence of machines.

THE ANCIENT LANGUAGE OF EMOTION

Emotions are undoubtedly an ancient part of the human mind. They probably originated long before language, as a way of giving meaning to preverbal thought. When language evolved, the expression of sensory data stored as memories became more precise. Communication with others also became much easier and more rapid. The brain could now use both language and emotion to interpret its storehouse of memories. The two probably worked in combination to provide people with a clearer understanding of their world. Both are ways the brain uses to understand and express the sensory data it stores as memories.

Memories, language and emotion are the three main components of thought. The first two are, of course, the product of learning and experience acquired through individual maturation. In contrast, at least some emotion seems to be present and functional at the time of birth. We have all witnessed children in the first hours of life display anger, fear, happiness, frustration, and pleasure in response to their environment. Some emotional development is obviously present, although it is probably far from full maturity. Many studies have also indicated that infants show a wide range of natural temperaments, suggesting that some aspect of our emotional nature is inherited and operating at birth. Perhaps these primitive displays of emotion are *instinctual-like* responses to the world. Could there be some *hard-wired* inherited mental circuitry that guides this behavior? There really seems to be no other reasonable possibility. We accept this explanation for behavior that appears to be purely instinctual. Is there reason to think that emotional responses might not also be passed on in hard-wired form? Certainly they manifest themselves before any appreciable learning can occur. Some emotion would seem almost certainly to be of inherited origin.

The origin of emotion has long been debated. As indicated earlier, there is reason to believe that some emotion is present at birth and therefore hereditary. If this subject is carefully examined, it seems doubtful that true emotion can be learned at all from others. Certainly behavior can be modeled and learned by emulation, but only the outward manifestations of emotion can be directly observed. The inward feeling that we sense is a very individual experience, which is not available through observation. By watching others, we certainly can learn when various emotions are appropriate and should be used. This learning process undoubtedly occurs as children grow and mature. This is, however, quite different from acquiring the inward feeling we know as the emotion. A person who had never experienced anger might recognize it in others but could not appreciate it emotionally. There might be a cognitive understanding, but the feeling itself would not be generated by its outward manifestations. It is easy to see how the use of an emotion might be observed in others and learned, but it is much more difficult to see how the inner feeling itself could be transmitted in this way. This would appear to be a subtle but important distinction, and suggests that emotions may have their origin in inheritance. This idea is further supported by the observation that children born deaf and dumb and those with severe mental retardation still display emotion, even though their ability to learn by observation may be grossly limited. In addition, autistic children, who may have normal intelligence, show a decreased ability to acquire and express emotion, despite a normal ability to learn.

DARWIN AND EMOTION

Charles Darwin also believed that the expression of emotion was inborn and had a definite survival value. During his travels, he noted that there were a great many similarities in the way people of different cultures expressed specific emotions. To investigate this further, he compared the emotional expression of children who had been blind from birth with that of normal children. If facial expressions and other behaviors were learned emotional responses, he reasoned that blind children should express emotion differently than those with sight. His observations and those of later investigators showed essentially no difference between the two groups (Eibl-Eibesfeldt, 1970; Thompson, 1941). Both blind and sighted children showed similar reactions in comparable situations. These findings strongly support the contention that much emotion is innate and functional at birth.

INHERITED EMOTION AND GENERALIZED KNOWLEDGE

From the preceding discussion, it seems at least plausible that some emotion is inherited rather than learned. Unlike the other two elements of thought, this component shows evidence of being at least partially present at birth. According to the overall hypothesis presented here, emotions exist only in physical association with the memories they define. Unlike some memories, emotions cannot exist alone. They must have an associated memory to be expressed when information is evaluated cognitively. As will be discussed later in this chapter, emotional activation can probably also occur in the apparent absence of conscious memory recall. In such cases, the matching and activation of generalized knowledge, which may not be perceived as memory in consciousness, may result in emotional experience.

It seems possible that over the millennia, some very stable and constant generalized knowledge has become hard-wired into neural circuitry and is passed from one generation to the next in unchanged form. This type of knowledge is, in essence, the wisdom of the ages and represents that small fraction of information that is critical for the survival of mankind and has remained true under all conditions of human existence. This type of knowledge constitutes our instincts and probably many other less-recognized behavioral patterns. It is via this route that emotions may be inherited. As hard-wired information is passed from one generation to the next, its associated emotion would also be transmitted. Once again, this emotion would represent the most stable interpretation for the generalized knowledge involved. It, too, would be established as the truest and most representative emotional response for the situations represented by generalized knowledge. It would literally be the most correct emotional interpretation, as determined over millions of years of experience. The idea that emotions are instinctual and arise from inherited, built-in circuitry is certainly not new (McDougall, 1910).

When an infant smiles or shows displeasure by crying, it is responding to some environmental cue that has undergone localization and matching with its store of hard-wired knowledge. In essence, it is reacting instinctively to its surroundings. It cries because countless children have cried before in similar circumstances. The emotion of displeasure has remained associated with the given situation and has become established as the most accurate and common interpretation through evolutionary time. All emotions it might express at this point are probably instinctive reactions to cues that match hard-wired generalized knowledge. Its expression of this emotion is the most appropriate interpretation, as established over time. In addition to the expression of emotion, this mechanism may be valid for all other forms of instinctual behavior. In other words, those behaviors we consider instinctual are also probably responses to various situations that are retained in generalized knowledge and passed from one generation to the next.

It is proposed here that the emotion displayed by infants is a form of generalized knowledge that has become stable over evolutionary time. It is similar, if not identical, to the type of information we commonly recognize as instinctual. It specifically consists of ancient memories of various general situations linked in association with their appropriate emotional responses. In this way, the child is born with the ability to interpret and react to a number of common environmental cues. This allows the infant to transmit its feelings in a crude way to its caregiver. At this point, the number of emotions available to the infant is probably limited to those that it can crudely project. The full range of adult responses is probably not yet fully developed.

As the infant matures, its bank of acquired memories grows and progresses toward generalized knowledge. At this point, many memories are probably imprinted in virgin neuronal structures, because little information is present to allow localization and matching with existing structures. The organization of new material into early generalized clusters would be actively occurring. Interpretation would be crude or nonexistent for many events recorded in memory. As indicated, some new memories would match hard-wired, generalized knowledge, allowing crude emotion to be expressed. Each new memory interpreted in this way would acquire the emotion released as an association. In effect, the emotional interpretation derived from hard-wired knowledge would be transferred to each new memory, and would therefore be available for interpretation of future events. Over time, emotion would be carried forward by this mechanism to many events stored as memory. The spread would parallel and accompany the general growth of knowledge. Emotion would be transferred forward over time from the original hardwired, generalized form present at birth to most of the memories acquired through experience. The basis for this process would, of course, be association. Any emotion used for interpretation would become linked with new memory and transferred forward in this way. This process would be continuous and occur throughout life. The basic pool of emotion present at birth would provide the seed by which this process would be initiated in each individual.

DIVERSITY OF EMOTION

The outward expression of emotion in human beings can take many forms. These commonly include changes in facial expression, body language, and verbal inflection. These, of course, have long been recognized as components of communication. In combination with language, they allow us to express our inward feelings to others. Certain emotions can be easily transmitted in this way. Joy, anger, and frustration, among others, are easily recognized. There are, however, many more emotions that are very subtle and only inwardly sensed. Actually the number of things that can be only felt and therefore defined as emotions is very large. Many of these may be experienced only as a vague, fleeting, inner awareness that provides us with understanding of a thought or situation. The following is a partial listing of common emotions. The grammatical form of each word was chosen so that it would be appropriate for the sentence "He or she is feeling _____." Such lists have been published by others (DeRivera, 1977).

Adequate • Affectionate • Agony • Alarmed • Altruistic • Amazed • Ambivalent • Anger • Annoyed • Anxious • Astonished

Bad • Belittled • Belligerent • Benevolent • Berated • Betrayed • Bitter • Bold • Bored • Brave • Burdened

Calm • Capable • Capricious • Charmed • Cheated • Cheerful •Clever • Competent • Comfortable • Competitive • Concerned •Confounded • Confused • Confident • Content • Cruel • Curious • Cursed

Deceitful • Degenerate • Delightful • Depressed • Desirous • Despondent • Despair • Destructive • Determined •

Different • Discontented • Dismayed • Dissatisfied • Distant • Distracted • Distraught • Disturbed • Dysphoric

Eager • Empathy • Empty • Enchanted • Energetic • Enthusiastic • Envious • Euphoric • Evil • Exasperated • Excited • Exhausted • Exhilarated

Fanciful • Fascinated • Fearful • Flustered • Foolish • Forlorn •Frantic • Friendly • Frustrated • Frightened • Free • Furious

Giddy • Generous • Glad • Glamorous • Good • Gracious • Great • Gregarious • Greedy • Grief • Guilty

Happy • Hateful • Helpful • Helpless • Homesick • Honest • Honored • Horrible • Hostile • Humble • Hurt • Hysterical

Indifferent • Infuriated • Inspired • Insulted • Intimidated • Isolated

Jealous • Joyous • Jaded

Kind • Kinship

Lazy • Lonely • Longing • Loyal • Lustful

Mad • Maudlin • Misunderstood • Mean • Mischievous • Miserly • Miserable

Naive • Naughty • Neglected • Nervous • Nice

Obsessed • Obstinate • Odd • Opposed • Ordinary • Overwhelmed

Pain • Panic • Paranoia • Peaceful • Pensive • Persecuted • Petrified • Pitiful • Pleasant • Pleasure • Pressured • Pretty • Powerful • Proud

Rage • Refreshed • Rejected • Relaxed • Relieved • Remorseful • Resentful • Resigned • Respectful • Restless • Rushed

Sad • Satisfied • Scared • Selfish • Sensual • Shocked • Silly •Sinful • Skeptical • Sneaky • Sorrowful • Spiteful • Startled • Strange • Stunned • Sure • Surprised • Sympathetic

Tempted • Tense • Terrible • Threatened • Tired • Troubled

Ugly • Uneasy • Useful • Urgency

Valuable • Victimized • Violent • Vicious • Vivacious • Vulnerable

Weak • Wicked • Wise • Wishful • Wonderful • Worried

The previous listing is presented to illustrate the great variety of emotions that can be experienced by the brain. They have been classified here as emotions, because they are not sensed verbally or as memories of physical reality. They are *truly felt* by the brain and, as such, might be described as mental sensations.

EMOTION AS A MENTAL LANGUAGE

Emotions seem to be the brain's way of expressing its immediate condition. This seems analogous to the body's use of pain and other tactile sensation as an indicator of physical status. Emotions, like physical sensation, must be experienced to be understood. There are no adequate words or images to describe pain to someone who has never experienced it. Like emotions, such sensations seem to be an ancient form of internal communication. Although external, physical manifestations of emotion can often be sensed by others, these entities probably originally arose as a form of internal mental language. In contrast, words may have evolved primarily as a rapid and direct form of external communication between people. By examining the numerous entries in the previous listing, it is obvious that the brain has a wide range of options by which to express itself on an internal level.

As indicated before, emotions seem to provide the driving impetus for thought. The type and quantity of emotion sensed by the brain at any time may determine and direct subsequent thinking. It is proposed that each thought that cycles through the brain undergoes localization and matching, as described. The interpretation derived in this way would be a blend of the individual component structures identified in this process. Each GMC overlapped by similar incoming data would add something to the resulting understanding by releasing its associated emotion. The final interpretation would therefore be a *blend of such emotions.* The ultimate feeling produced would be sensed as a combination of component emotions. This process is probably the origin of the many and varied emotional states of which we are aware.

PRIMAL EMOTION

At birth, there are probably a discrete number of primary emotions linked with the inherited, generalized knowledge that has been passed forward through evolutionary time. Events that match such information would stimulate the release of this emotion and then become linked in association with the new memory that is stored. It is likely that mixed interpretations eventually arose as memory stores grew and understanding became more sophisticated. Through this process, primary emotion probably became integrated or blended, allowing new situations to be more specifically defined. Many combinations of primal emotion may have arisen in this way and became stored in memory to serve as a reference for future events.

It should be noted that the affect theory, which was originally proposed by Tomkins in 1962 and 1963, also predicts that a limited number of emotions or affects are present at birth. In this hypothesis, nine innate affects are described, two of which represent positive emotions, one a neutral emotion, and six that are negative. This theory, however, assumes that emotion is not initially linked with memory but acquires such associations as a consequence of life experience. In other words, no inherited, generalized memory is present to initially guide the expression and spread of such primal emotion.

THE STRUCTURE OF EMOTIONAL LANGUAGE

Perhaps it would be helpful to briefly comment on how a nonverbal mental language based on emotion might be structured. We can speculate that inherited, generalized knowledge is collectively composed of numerous neural patterns, which encode crude identifying information about a wide range of situations and circumstances. To each individual structure, one or more emotions would be associated, which would be triggered when the main complex was activated in response to incoming data. As discussed before, emotion associated in this way would provide a form of interpretation for this inherited information. It is reasonable to assume that those structures with the highest degree of associative integrity would correlate with situations important for survival. Such complexes would constitute what we commonly recognize as drives and instincts. A great many complexes would also exist, which would have weaker or less well-associated structures. Such complexes would represent more routine and less threatening situations, and would be much more difficult to recognize for the scientific observer.

We can speculate that an infant would initially respond to a given situation, which matched a neural structure within its store of generalized knowledge, with emotion only. As a consequence, the infants mother would initiate some action appropriate for this display of emotion. For example, a hungry, crying infant might be fed, or one who was smiling and contented might be kissed and held. In this way, the mother would eliminate or possibly prolong the emotion that was produced by the original situation. As a consequence of repeating this process over time, new learning in the infant would occur. It would eventually learn those events that would eliminate unpleasant emotion for a given situation, as well as those that might perpetuate any positive emotion that might be produced. We can speculate that the neural structures encoding such newly acquired learning would associate with the original, generalized knowledge–emotion complex. When the original situation was again encountered, activation of the corresponding generalized knowledge structure and its associated emotion would lead to activation of this learned remedy or action. Through this associative process, the child would learn that eating would eliminate hunger or that smiling would produce a favorable response in his or her mother. In a like manner, many other generalized situations paired with emotion would gradually acquire association from experience. In older children, such new learning might be acquired through experimental trial and error rather than from direct contact with their caregiver. Such learning would continue throughout life and the original, generalized knowledge–emotion complexes might grow very large and complex through the addition of new associated information. Through this simple associative process, a child might eventually learn a wide range of behavior that would eliminate or in some cases prolong various emotions evoked when generalized knowledge was activated. It is conceivable that the child's actions would eventually become completely directed by such emotional influences. At this point, a form of nonverbal emotional language would be in place. A child would act and react to life situations based on this neural storehouse of memories and associated emotion. In such a system, behavior would be somewhat automatic in that no reflective analysis utilizing an inner verbal language or other cognition would be necessary. Learned actions would be initiated almost reflexively in response to the activation of generalized knowledge and its interpretative emotion. Of course, the ultimate goal of this process would be to eliminate, modify, or extend the original emotion that was stimulated. In effect, emotion would drive learned behavior to maintain a current emotional state or produce a change in it. Such a system would constitute an emotional language employed by preverbal children and many animal forms. This process would essentially be noncognitive in that it could operate in the complete absence of mental analysis or reflection.

Through the aging and maturation process, we can speculate that inherited, generalized knowledge complexes would become more complex as new learned behavior, capable of influencing the original expression of emotion, were added. Verbal language would gradually be incorporated as sounds became associated with objects and concepts. Eventually, the level of complexity would become so great that true cognitive reflection, utilizing an inner form of verbal thought, would become possible. This new form of mental communication would be built on the older, nonverbal language developed earlier but would probably never completely replace it. This seems evident from observing our thinking. There are times we can be very reasonable and analytical in our decisions, and at others, emotion seems to rule, and behavior seems almost reflexive. This suggests the presence of both systems, which can operate at different times and levels of complexity.

These concepts are indirectly supported by the work of others who have speculated that emotion can be expressed in the absence of true cognition. In 1993, in *Psychological Review*, Izard argued convincingly that there are three noncognitive ways in which emotion can be produced. The first of these involves the activation of emotion through chemical or electrical stimulation of appropriate brain regions and is referred as the *neural system*. As Izard pointed out, drugs such as antidepressants that affect neurotransmitter systems can produce changes in mood and emotional experience. In addition, drugs such as cocaine and amphetamines, which are known to interact with the transmission of neural impulses, can produce almost immediate changes in emotional expression, without the direct involvement of cognition. These ideas are consistent with the overall conceptualization presented here that emotions arise from neural structures through factors that influence neurotransmission.

Izard's second form of noncognitive emotional activation is referred to as the *sensorimotor system*. It is proposed that emotional activation occurs in response to muscle activity mediated by proprioceptive and other sensory structures located outside the central nervous system. Central to this proposal is the observation that facial and postural movement can often initiate emotional experience that appears to be independent of cognitive influence. It seems possible that the physical movements involved in the creation of numerous facial expressions could be encoded in the form of generalized knowledge that is present at birth. Activation of such a complex would produce discrete facial movement and release of the associated emotion. For example, joy may be associated with neural complexes that contain generalized information about smiling. In a like manner, sadness and distress may be elicited by a frown. Such emotional expression would be automatic, in that it may be evoked by pure physical movement, in the absence of significant cognition.

The last form of noncognitive emotional activation described by Izard involves *motivational systems* such as drives and instincts. As indicated in an earlier paragraph, these entities may actually be inherited forms of generalized knowledge that are strongly associated with motivating emotion. Through activation of such a complex in response to a matching situation, secondary associated structures coding for compensatory behavior may also receive stimulation and undergo activation. As explained before, this would represent a somewhat automatic, noncognitive attempt to change or in some way influence the original emotion. The ideas presented here support Izard's contention that emotion can be produced in noncognitive systems that involve motivational factors.

The notion that at least some emotion can be elicited through noncognitive routes is directly supported by the elucidation of subcortical neural pathways that mediate fear conditioning. This work will be discussed under the Amygdala section in Chapter 7.

EMOTIONAL EXPRESSION DURING THOUGHT

As thoughts cycle through the brain, each is evaluated, and emotion is released, which contributes to the dominant emotional tone. If a certain issue is being considered, this process may continue for some time, and many ideas may be examined. As various aspects of a given issue pass through the brain, a certain feeling may be established by the cumulative emotion that is produced. The brain may sense satisfaction, anxiety, creativity, or any of many possible emotions. The train of thought may largely be guided by these feelings. If anxiety is experienced, perhaps there will be a shift to other aspects of the issue, which, in some way, might produce a more favorable emotion. Alternately, the brain might try to find a way to circumvent the problems leading to this emotion. If the issue being considered produces a pleasurable feeling, more time and attention might be invested on this subject. The key to this process seems to involve a form of feedback in which the brain strives to generate and maintain favorable emotion. Thoughts may wander in many directions until an acceptable emotion is sensed. If a line of thought produces unpleasant emotion, this may serve as impetus for a change in direction.

Of course, thinking is probably not simply a matter of generating pleasurable emotion. In a more general sense, it might be described as a way of finding the most acceptable way to deal with the problems encountered in life. The applicability of any solution will be judged by the type of emotion generated. This might involve pleasurable feelings or any number of emotions specifying an option. With the wide range of emotions available to the brain, virtually any response would seem possible. Almost any situation could undergo evaluation and be expressed in an appropriate emotional manner. It should also be noted that many emotions we experience during thought are subtle and may go almost unnoticed. They may exist only as brief, fleeting, and barely perceptible evidence of emotional thought.

Memories have been postulated to exist as clusters of neurons electrically connected by discrete patterns of neurotransmission. These structures are further organized into larger units, which are extensively overlapped and interconnected, reflecting the various relationships present. In this way, many memories are physically linked via their natural association in experience. Emotions also seem to exist in association with these structures. Evidence for this comes from the observation that the recall of a specific memory will often result in the release of the same emotion that was present at the time of memory storage. It seems probable that these relationships would also be established and maintained by specific modifications in the ionic channels linking the involved entities. But how might emotions be physically described? Do they exist as neuronal clusters, as postulated for memories, or might they involve the release of specific types or combinations of neurotransmitters from the neurons of activated memory structures? There would appear to be many ways emotion might be encoded within the brain. Perhaps some older observations might be of value here.

THE BIOLOGY OF EMOTION

It has long been recognized that certain brain regions seem to be specifically involved in the expression of emotion. Injuries to structures of the limbic system or frontal cortex often produce profound disruptions in the expression of emotion. Because of this, many investigators have speculated that there may be emotional centers within the brain that mediate the various feelings we experience. This idea has received some criticism because of the large number of centers that would be necessary for the great variety of emotions at our disposal. As suggested here, the numerous mental sensations we experience may result from the combination of a few basic emotions. Perhaps emotional centers do exist for these dominant or major emotions, and through their combination the lesser emotions are generated. Such centers might have numerous, widespread synaptic connections linking them to memory storage areas throughout the brain. Any given center might form active association linkages with thousands of individual memories. Activation of such a memory would produce a subsequent flow of neurotransmission to the emotional center, resulting in its entry into consciousness. Of course, this is the same process that would occur with each of the memory's other associations. An emotional center activated in this way would result in the perception of an emotion by the brain. A given memory might have association linkages to several primary emotional centers and their simultaneous stimulation might result in the generation of numerous blended emotions. The exact feeling produced by a thought or sensory perception would correspond to the combination of centers activated during the interpretive process.

The idea that emotional centers exist within the brain is supported by work begun by Olds and Milner at McGill University in 1954. These investigators showed that rats with an electrode placed in the hypothalamus appeared to experience pleasure upon electrical stimulation. If allowed to control the rate of self-stimulation by pressing a bar, rats would often maintain rates of 100 impulses per minute for hours, until completely exhausted. Food, sex, and other normally pleasurable activities were frequently ignored. From these experiments it was concluded that electrical stimulation of the hypothalamus was intensely pleasurable for the rat.

Since this initial work, pleasure centers have been found in many animal species, including man. In addition, such centers have also been identified in all levels of the brain, from the medulla oblongata to the cerebral cortex. Centers have also been identified that seem to produce only negative or punishing emotion. These effects were initially reported by Delgado, Roberts, and Miller in 1954. In other studies utilizing human participants, feelings of anxiety, isolation, fear, and abandonment were also produced by stimulation of a number of brain regions. Taken together, these data support the idea that discrete centers may exist within the brain that mediate the expression of emotion. Memories may become electrically linked with one or more of these centers during the storage process, as described earlier. The subsequent localization and activation of such a memory would result in the transmission of energy to its associations, as well as to any linked emotional centers. The memory and its emotional interpretation would thus be specified and sensed together in consciousness. In this way, the emotion released would be immediately present to influence further thought. As proposed here, the attainment of an appropriate emotional state may be the driving force behind the direction taken by thought.

MOOD AS CUMULATIVE EMOTION IN CONSCIOUSNESS

As indicated, emotions may be transferred from one entity to the next during the interpretation of new data. An incoming piece of sensory information or a thought passing through consciousness may undergo evaluation by identification of similar stored memories, and the emotion released may become reassociated. In this way, the new data would acquire the emotional interpretation of one or more older memories. This would allow past experience to contribute to current understanding. Most emotion released in this process is subtle and would not be experienced as a separate, individual feeling. In many cases, it may be hardly perceptible to the conscious brain. It would serve its purpose and rapidly dissipate. This would seem to be the case when we deal with most routine, daily matters. In contrast, some memories are associated with intense emotion. These may be issues of particular significance, and their memories reflect this by the type and quantity of associated emotion. Their recall during the interpretation process may produce a significant level of emotional release, which is easily sensed in consciousness.

The emotional tone established in this way may linger within the brain long after the associated thought has vanished. We have all experienced situations in which this has occurred. An argument with our spouse at breakfast may leave us in a bad mood for the rest of the day, or the feeling produced by some pleasurable event may remain with us for hours after the thought itself has dissipated. Strong emotion seems to have this unique quality. Once experienced, these intense feelings may linger in the background for quite some time without any conscious effort. This *emotional glow* may persist and color all our subsequent activities for as long as it endures. It may subtly influence our thinking and actions. Our decisions, activities, and relationships with others may be slightly altered. In essence, the way we do things may be influenced somewhat because of the prevailing emotional tone.

The dominant emotional tone described may also be produced from the cumulative effects of smaller quantities of emotion. Large, obvious bursts of emotion may be only one way this background tone is generated. The continuous release of smaller quantities of emotion during routine interpretation, or the activation of generalized knowledge, as described before, may eventually be sensed as a dominant feeling. For example, the many, small, cumulative irritations of a day may eventually generate an overall sense of frustration and increased irritability. In a like manner, the effects of several small pleasurable events may add together over time to produce a pleasing emotional tone. In most cases, the

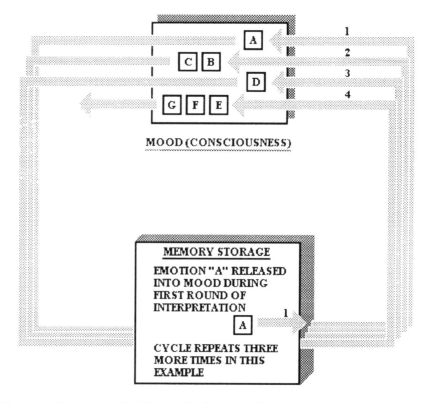

Figure 5.1 It is proposed that the mood is the cumulative perception of emotion released during the interpretation of sensory data and/or the cycling of thought. In this figure, four interpretative rounds (labeled 1–4) are shown, in which emotions A–G are released during the activation of memory and sensed in consciousness. Note that, for clarity, the memory structures themselves are not shown. It is assumed that the intensity of an emotion begins to fade as soon as it enters consciousness and, therefore, some entities in this mood may be strong, whereas others may be barely perceptible. It is also assumed that moods are sensed as a blend of all emotions present in consciousness at any given time.

prevailing tone may be somewhat neutral, reflecting a balanced mixture of both positive and negative emotion. The ability of emotion to linger within the brain seems to allow it to mix and be sensed cumulatively. In this way, both intense and subtle emotion may each contribute to our dominant emotional tone. This constant background noise is what we commonly refer to as mood.

Mood may be described as a prevailing emotional tone that lingers in the background of consciousness. It frames and influences our thoughts, mental activities, and subsequent actions. It seems to be the cumulative product of the emotional release arising from our constant cognitive and noncognitive interpretations of the world. As such, it seems to be a general measure of our emotional status at any given time. In essence, it reflects the events of our lives as we perceive them. Each time emotion is released during the interpretive process, it blends with the mood, changing its overall character somewhat. In this way, the interpretation of routine memories contributes to the general mood. The emotion released during the interpretation of an individual memory is specific for the single event that triggered the process. In contrast, mood is the result of many individual interpretations and, as such, can be viewed as a measure of overall emotional status at any given point in time. The accumulation of emotion in the mood from the ongoing interpretation of data is illustrated in Figure 5.1.

EMOTION AS A FORM OF INTERPRETATION

When an individual memory is triggered, its emotional release provides an interpretation based on past experience. The current event stimulating this process would thus be viewed in the same way as the similar, original event depicted in memory and used for interpretation. By itself, an interpretation generated in this way would seem to be only partially complete.

The pairing of a current event with a similar one from the past would only provide information that was relevant at the time the reference memory was stored. In other words, an interpretation such as this would only tell us about a similar situation that may have occurred years before. Its relevancy to the present situation could not be established without further information. This difficulty can be eliminated if we assume that the emotion from the interpretation is mixed with the mood and evaluated in this context. Older information would thus be integrated with the current emotional tone so that it might have more applicability to the immediate situation. It would be judged not as an isolated piece of data from the past, but in relationship to the present situation. It seems possible that this is a critical function of the mood.

In some situations the mood would act as a buffer for emotion released during the interpretive process. If the mood were composed predominately of pleasant emotion, the release of negative feelings through interpretation might not alter the overall emotional tone significantly. The brain might experience some negative feeling, but perhaps not to the same extent as if the mood had been neutral or dysphoric. Obviously the memory yielding the negative emotion might be seen in a less significant way than was the original similar event providing the interpretation. Any subsequent action or thought would, in turn, also be influenced by the particular interpretation produced by this blend of emotions. This illustrates the general process by which old information is combined with new to reflect current relevance. Were the released emotion not integrated into the mood, its interpretation would be exactly as experienced in the past, which might not be appropriate for the present situation. The mood may allow released emotion to be tempered with our current emotional tone for a more relevant interpretation. A mechanism for this is proposed in the next chapter.

It seems likely that every new memory that is stored incorporates some of the existing emotional tone as an association. In fact, each thought we experience, or each old memory that is recalled into consciousness, probably associates with some of the emotional context provided by the mood. As indicated, this may serve to frame each new memory with a current reference and, in a like manner, may update older, recalled memories. Storing specific emotions with memories may also serve another important function. As associated components of larger memories, emotions may be able to participate in the localization process. As proposed, many different emotions may be generated by combining a relatively small number of basic emotions. A primary emotion, or combination of such entities, may act in concert with other associations in the search for specific memories. This is a concept of immense importance and will be further developed in the next chapter.

OVERVIEW OF EMOTION

In this chapter, a theory of emotion has been presented. It is based upon the premise that this elusive quality exists in association with memories. When a thought or incoming sensory perception is interpreted by comparison with existing memories, there is a release and transfer of emotion to the new memories generated. In this way, new information is evaluated in light of past experience, and the emotional interpretation derived is stored in association with the new entity to provide a reference for future evaluation.

It has been suggested here that certain basic emotions are inherited are passed from one memory to the next throughout our lives. Original emotion might thus be viewed as a master blueprint that guides us throughout life. It is well known that emotion governs many of our autonomic responses in various situations by stimulating the peripheral release of catecholamine. On a central level, emotions may play an equally important role by driving thought and subsequent action. They may also serve as markers that allow us to distinguish important memories from those that are perhaps more trivial.

It is postulated that a relatively small number of basic, pure emotions exist. These are physically represented by specialized brain regions, which are connected to perhaps hundreds of thousands of individual memories by synaptic connections. A given memory may exist in association with one or several of these centers. When a memory is activated, it triggers its associated memories as well as emotional centers. Emotion associated with the memory is thus sensed by the brain. If the memory is linked with more than one emotional center, a mixed feeling will result. In this way many lesser (blended) emotions can be generated.

The interpretation of thoughts and incoming data is essentially an ongoing process. The emotion released during this process can accumulate and linger within the brain to produce an emotional background. This is perceived as the prevailing mood and can influence subsequent thoughts, activities, and memory storage. The interdependent relationship of memory and emotion will be discussed in the next chapter.

State-Dependency
and Emotion

Under most circumstances, memory recall appears to be a spontaneous process that requires little obvious conscious effort. As we engage in thought, cues arising from previous cognitive activity or sensory perception trigger a continuous stream of memories that pass through consciousness. A careful examination of this process suggests that some memories seem to be readily activated under a wide variety of circumstances, whereas others appear to require more specific conditions. For example, in some cases, remembering seems to be strongly dependent upon reproducing the conditions that existed during storage of the original events. When circumstances are different, recall may be inefficient or fail completely. When the particular situation is again reproduced, the ability to recall the involved memories may return. For obvious reasons, this very interesting effect has been termed *context- or state-dependent memory*. It may underlie a number of psychological conditions such as repression, multiple personality disorder, functional amnesia, and other forms of dissociative phenomena. Despite its obvious importance in psychiatry, it may play an even more significant and central role in non-pathological mental processes. This idea will be developed here.

EMOTION IN MEMORY LOCALIZATION

The phenomenon of context- or state-dependent memory suggests that the storage or recall of a memory may be heavily dependent upon the learning environment. Work in this area has demonstrated that memory recall is most efficient when the conditions present during the original learning session are duplicated at the time of recall. This effect can largely be explained if we assume that a memory's emotional component plays an essential role in its localization. This point can best be demonstrated by examining some of the work that has been done in this area.

STATE-DEPENDENCY IN LEARNING

State-dependent learning has been observed under many naturally occurring circumstances and has been experimentally verified in several ways. In 1969, Goodwin, Powell, Bremer, Hoine, and Stern studied the role of state-dependency in heavy users of alcohol. They cite examples of alcoholics who, when sober, were unable to remember where they hid alcohol or money while in an intoxicated state. When they again became drunk, the memories of these secret hiding places returned. In other words, successful recall of these memories was dependent upon reestablishing the original mental state present during their storage. This is just one example illustrating the apparent interdependence of mental state and memory.

In other experiments, Overton (1964) found evidence of state-dependent learning in rats treated with sodium pentobarbital. This effect was much like that seen in alcoholics. Tasks learned in the drugged state did not transfer to the nondrugged state and vice versa. In addition, he showed that the effect was dose-dependent (i.e., the greater the dosage of medication, the larger was the decremental effect on memory between the two states). Since this work, state-dependent learning and memory recall have been demonstrated with a variety of drugs and species. Much of this work is reviewed in a book by Ho, Richards, and Chute (1978).

STATE-DEPENDENCY WITHOUT DRUGS

State-dependent learning can also be demonstrated without the use of drugs. In 1975, Godden and Baddeley used divers as subjects to produce the same effect. These individuals were asked to learn a list of words either on shore or under water at a depth of about 6 meters. Recall was tested either in the same environment or in the opposite one. Those who learned the word list under water showed a 40% drop in retention when tested on the shore, as compared with those who originally learned on shore. The same occurred for the other experimental group when tested in the opposite environment. Once again, learning and recall were interpreted as dependent upon the context or the mental state involved. In a subsequent experiment, these subjects were given a recognition test in which they were asked simply to identify original words in a new list consisting of both presented and nonpresented words. No state-dependent decrement in recall was detected under these conditions. This was interpreted as evidence that context-dependency is a *retrieval effect*. The presentation of an original word itself in the second list was felt to be a sufficient cue for recall. Under these conditions, contextual associations may not have been necessary for retrieval.

MOOD AS A FACTOR IN THE LOCALIZATION OF MEMORIES

In other experiments performed by Bower, Monteiro, and Gilligan (1978), the learner's emotional status was found to produce state-dependent memory. In other words, the mood state itself present during learning seemed to act as a contextual reference for this effect. Under hypnosis, human subjects were influenced to feel happy while learning one list of words and sad while learning another. Retention was tested either in the same mood as present during learning or the opposite. Lists learned and recalled in the same mood state averaged a 78% retention rate. Those learned in one state and recalled in the other produced only a 47% retention rate. These authors concluded that mood can act as a distinctive context, which can become attached to newly learned material and influence subsequent searches for that material in memory.

In subsequent studies by Bower (1981; Bower, Gilligan, & Monteiro, 1981), the state-dependency of memory was again tested using a *mood induction* hypnotic procedure to alter the emotional status of subjects during learning sessions. Once again, a *mood-congruency* effect was noted (i.e., the mood exhibited during recall seemed to facilitate the recall of memories learned under similar emotional conditions). A failure to replicate these findings (Hasher, Rose, Zacks, Sanft, & Doren, 1985) has produced some controversy as to whether these effects occur regularly in normal subjects. It was suggested that the mood-induction procedure used in these studies may have produced inconsistent results. The mechanism for state-dependency, which will be presented in this chapter, suggests that this phenomenon may be subtle and difficult to detect with regularity in subjects without major psychiatric pathology.

STATE-DEPENDENCY IN PATHOLOGICAL CONDITIONS

It is a common observation among psychiatric workers that patients with severe depression are generally unable to recall memories with a happy or positive emotional connotation. Such memories just seem to be unavailable for reference in the presence of the severely dysphoric mood that characterizes this disorder. Formal studies have also confirmed this general observation. In 1981, Clark and Teasdale examined the types of memories recalled by depressed patients who displayed mood swings. During relative positive periods, more happy than unhappy memories were recalled. When deeper depression became dominate, unpleasant memory recall seemed to fill consciousness. In 1975, Lloyd and Lishman observed that the time necessary to recall negative or unpleasant experiences decreased as depression became more intense in their study group. Other studies have produced similar results (Williams & Broadbent, 1986). A review of this subject was published by Williams, Watts, Macleod, and Mathews in 1988. In a related study, the effect of anxiety on memory recall was examined (Burke & Mathews, 1992). When patients who were judged to be clinically anxious were presented with neutral cues, they were found to recall more anxiety-related memories than a control group of nonanxious subjects. These data suggest that state-dependent effects may be prominent in some forms of psychiatric illness. This will be further considered in subsequent chapters that deal with mood disorders.

STATE-DEPENDENCY AND MEMORY RECALL

The hypothesis presented here is based upon the thesis that an associative relationship between mood and memory exists, which can influence recall in normal as well as pathological states. As stated before, each new thought or perception that passes through consciousness may incorporate emotion from the mood as it becomes stored in memory. This emotion may therefore serve as a contextual reference, which becomes associated with each new memory. In other words, the dominant mood may mark each new memory with emotion that can later be used during the localization process. If the individual is under the influence of alcohol or other drugs, this should strongly influence the dominant mood. Memories stored in a drugged state should therefore incorporate a contextual mood reflecting this altered emotional state. Each memory stored under these conditions should thus possess a unique associated emotion reproducible only through intoxication. If emotions function as do other associations in the localization process, the retrieval of a specific memory should be dependent to some extent upon reexperiencing the same emotion at the time of recall. Emotion would therefore serve as any retrieval cue participating with other associations providing energy for activation of the memory in question. In the absence of intoxication, this cue from the mood would not be present, and recall would depend upon whatever other cues to the memory might be present. In many cases, this might be insufficient to produce recall. Thus, the sober alcoholic might not have an important emotional cue necessary to fully trigger the memories of things done while intoxicated. The absence of a specific emotion may produce retrieval failure in exactly the same way as might any other missing cue. Whenever any critical stimulus is absent, an important associated part of the memory may not be activated.

The same principles may apply to the state-dependent effects noted in the diving experiments. In each case, learning was accomplished in a different physical environment. The elements of each setting should have produced a unique emotional interpretation during the matching and localization process. Each set of emotions released in this way should have combined with the predominant emotional tone to produce a mood specific for the given physical surroundings. In effect, a different mood was established in each setting, corresponding to prior experiences in similar settings. Learning was therefore associated with the emotional context present in each circumstance. When retrieval was attempted in a different context, an important cue for the localization of the memory was not available. When recognition of a previously presented word was the only requirement, sufficient information was presented so that the emotional association was not necessary for retrieval. As postulated, for any memory to be localized, a sufficient number of cues must be present for it to be completely specified.

STATE-DEPENDENCY AS A FUNCTION OF EMOTION

The phenomenon of state-dependent memory may therefore be a function of the contextual emotion associated with memory during storage. If the same or similar emotional state is not present during recall, an important retrieval cue may be missing. Under these conditions, recall may be difficult or even impossible. It seems likely that all our memories become associated, to one degree or another, with contextual emotion from the mood. This seems unavoidable, considering that all of our thoughts and activities are framed in the prevailing mood of the moment. These concepts may also help to explain the various types of memory loss observed in amnesia. This will be considered in the next chapter.

STATE-DEPENDENCY AND MEMORY RETRIEVAL

The hypothesis presented suggests that state-dependent retrieval deficits may result from a mismatch in the current mood and the emotional association of the memory. In the examples presented here, an extreme interdependency of emotion and memory is easily observable. Under normal, daily conditions, state-dependency may also produce effects that are important but perhaps less dramatic. Retrieval effects probably operate whenever a memory is recalled but may only become obvious during unusual or pathological mood states. For example, severely depressed patients are often unable to recall even a single happy prior event in their lives. This may be an example of state-dependent recall failure, which may retard recovery from this illness. In nondepressed individuals, state-dependent memory effects may be less obvious but just as important. This will be addressed in subsequent paragraphs.

STATE-DEPENDENCY AS A DIRECTOR OF THOUGHT

It seems possible that the selective bias imposed by various mood states may control memory recall and, thereby, influence day-to-day thinking in nonpathological situations. This is certainly an intriguing possibility. Such a mechanism might help to explain the interdependency of emotion and thought that seems to exist. In effect, this process may explain the apparent ability of emotion to drive and direct thought. Perhaps state-dependency is only the obvious portion of a more general underlying mechanism influencing mental activity. Let us consider these questions in more detail. A brief review of prior concepts might be helpful before presenting this idea in full.

MOOD AS CUMULATIVE EMOTION

As suggested earlier, the mood seems to represent a cumulative mixture of emotions derived from recent interpretations. Each thought or incoming sensory perception that undergoes evaluation yields some emotion that contributes to this background tone. In this way, the mood reflects the sum of recent mental activity. The emotions that compose the mood may linger within the brain for minutes to hours and cumulatively influence all interpretations that occur. In this way, recalled memories may be provided with a current emotional relevance, as discussed before. This may be one of the chief purposes of the mood.

EMOTIONS AS ASSOCIATIONS OF MEMORIES

Emotions seem to exist within the brain as associations of memories. In this role, they seem to function as do all associations in the process of memory localization. Unlike other associations, emotions are not derived from external perception. These entities are triggered from memories during the interpretation process, become part of the mood, and can recombine with subsequent data passing through consciousness. In effect, each thought cycling through the brain, or each piece of new information acquired through sensory perception, becomes associated with the prevailing emotional tone, as well as with emotion released from those structures to which it corresponds during the matching process. A new memory will thus obtain emotion from two sources. Emotion from the mood will provide current contextual significance, and emotion released from identified and overlapped structures will convey past meaning. In this way, the new memory will have emotional associations that not only reflect the past but are also relevant to the present.

Consider a thought entering consciousness. It may have arisen from several memories or partial memories combined in consciousness during a previous cycle. On its passage through this domain, such a thought should acquire new emotions from the prevailing mood. In this way, its meaning would become slightly altered, requiring another evaluation. The thought and its new emotional associations would then be shuttled back into the unconscious interpretive areas for another round of matching and localization. A new interpretation would emerge, reflecting the addition of any emotion from the mood. Of course, additional cycles may occur, but if the mood does not change, the interpretation should remain the same, and the process should reach equilibrium for that given thought. In other words, a stable, cumulative interpretation reflecting any meaning derived from the original matched memories, combined with that from the current mood, would result.

The combining of thoughts and emotion in consciousness is really not a new concept to this hypothesis. It appears to be exactly analogous to the process described earlier, by which memories or partial memories

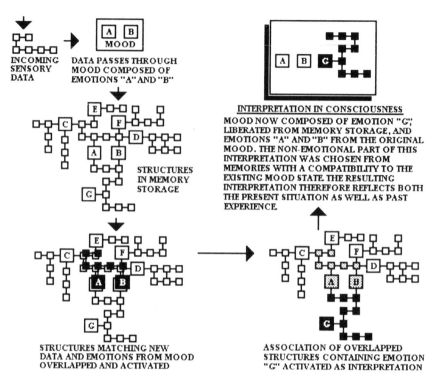

Figure 6.1 This figure illustrates how emotion from the mood can influence the localization and interpretation of memories corresponding to new sensory data. Incoming information is shown passing through the mood, where it associates with emotions A and B. These were deposited in the mood during previous interpretive rounds and, as such, reflect issues of current concern. Localization and overlapping of matching structures occur and, as a result, the associated structure is activated as the interpretation for original data. In this way, new information is understood in current contextual terms. In this illustration, emotions A and B serve to specify which of the four possible memories associated with the overlapped structure will be activated. If the original mood had been composed of other emotions, a different memory would have been localized and activated. In this way, the mood may impart current relevancy by influencing the selection of interpretation. Emotion G, which was liberated from memory storage during the interpretive process, is shown entering the mood and provides the memory part of the interpretation with meaning from the past. The final understanding of the incoming sensory data therefore reflects current relevancy as well as earlier experience.

are recombined to generate new thoughts. Both situations utilize the mixing of associations to generate entities with new meanings for the brain. The process of emotional and memory mixing probably occurs simultaneously on each round of cognitive activity. As indicated before, the pairing of previously unrelated associations seems to be a main function of consciousness.

MOOD AS A SOURCE OF EMOTIONAL ASSOCIATIONS

As indicated, thoughts passing through consciousness acquire new emotional associations from the mood. In essence, the new thought will gain emotional associations from recent mental activity, which may alter its overall meaning somewhat. This appears to be a way of updating older memories with current contextual emotion, as described earlier. The participation of these new emotional associations in the subsequent localization process should allow recent mental activity to be integrated into the resulting interpretation. Emotions from the mood probably serve as additional retrieval cues, selectively influencing which memories will be matched and localized. A specific combination of emotional cues, acquired from the mood, may match and partially activate those memories that originally contributed these emotions to the mood in the recent past. If the current thought contained other associations that also correspond to the earlier memories, the older structure may receive sufficient energy to become activated as a whole and thus, become part of the current interpretation. Figure 6.1 illustrates how emotions from the mood can influence the localization process, and how emotion from the past can mix with that from the mood to produce an interpretation with current relevancy.

EMOTION IN THE MOOD MAY DETERMINE
THE DIRECTION OF NEW THOUGHT

Because of the arrangement described, the emotional content present in the mood may selectively influence which memories are recalled into consciousness. Because mood is a reflection of recent events, those memories with the most current relevance will be selectively chosen for localization. Memories without current emotional reference in the mood may also be recalled, but they would require sufficient stimulation from the new thought by itself. In other words, enough nonemotional cues would need to be present within the thought to specify the memory, because no emotional associations from the mood would be matched. In this way, the mood seems to provide a bridge from recent mental activity to those thoughts under current evaluation. Such a process should focus our field of mental reference and allow emotion from the mood to determine the direction of new thought.

A mechanism by which emotions may influence thought has been proposed. In this way, the current emotional state may direct thinking so that relevant thoughts are preferentially retrieved. Each thought entering consciousness would be modified by the addition of new emotional associations from the mood. When the thought was sent back for unconscious interpretation, those memories most closely matching emotional cues from the mood and the associations of the new thought would be selectively activated. In this way, the current emotional status would produce the preferential recall of recent memories, which would contribute to the new interpretation. This system may prevent inappropriate thoughts from being generated and allow us to maintain continuity in thinking. This probably explains why it is easier to remember sad thoughts when our mood is predominantly dysphoric, or why we may readily become angry at small irritations if the events of the day have been unpleasant. Any emotion that becomes part of the prevailing mood should be capable of influencing subsequent thought in the manner described. This mechanism is the basis for the contention that emotion is the ultimate driver of thought.

STATE-DEPENDENCY AS A WIDESPREAD MENTAL PHENOMENON

The mechanism just postulated may represent a subtle expression of the dramatic state-dependent memory effects described by others. In essence, the well-known manifestations of this phenomenon may represent only the tip of the iceberg. The underlying principles may be much more widespread and represent a general mental process central to the flow of thought itself. The emotional composition of the mood probably influences all interpretations by producing selective memory recall. In turn, interpretations may cumulatively determine which emotions are added to the mood. The cyclic interdependency existing in this system may serve to maintain continuity in thought. The proposed mechanism would seem to provide a plausible basis by which this might be accomplished.

MOOD AND SHORT-TERM MEMORY

To better understand the mechanism proposed, it might be helpful to realize that the retention of thoughts in short-term memory seems analogous to the storage of emotions in the mood. Both mental entities serve as reservoirs in consciousness for emotional or factual-type data evoked from memory storage. In this way information can be temporally sequestered, so that it can actively participate in the generation of thought. From these pools of data, new thoughts will be constructed. Because both sources of information were generated by recent mental activity, the focus of new thought would be consistent with preceding ideas. In other words, by building thoughts from items held in the short-term memory and combining them with emotions from the mood, new thoughts should reflect recent mental activity. One idea should follow another in a logical, related manner.

DIRECTIONAL GUIDANCE FOR THOUGHT FROM THE MOOD

Any memory in storage may have a large number of other memories linked in association. Theoretically, many possible combinations of associations could be activated and follow the original memory in thought. In other words, thinking could potentially take many directions without some active guidance. It seems reasonable that the system proposed provides directional input for thought by selectively determining which combination of available associations might be activated in a given circumstance. The associations chosen should be those that correspond most closely with the ideas present in recent thought. In effect, the state-dependent mechanism proposed would provide specific direction for the movement of thought. In the absence of this guidance, thinking might still follow gross lines of association, but a general focus of ideas might be absent. Thinking might resemble the mental activity seen in dreams or the rambling confusion of a delirium. One association might still lead to another, but the process might be so tangential that little useful information could be generated. The mechanism proposed would allow those associations relevant to the issues at hand to be chosen from the many associated entities that might be potentially available.

To better understand how state-dependency may influence thought, let us examine a hypothetical situation. Assume the current mood is composed of emotions A, B, C and D. These four emotions would be, of course, sensed cumulatively and perceived as a single, blended feeling. A perception entering the senses would combine with these emotions as it passed through consciousness on the way to unconscious matching and localization. All such emotions acquired from the mood would serve as retrieval cues, along with nonemotional cues from the perception itself. As a result, all stored memories associated with one or more of these four emotions would receive some activation energy. The compatibility of such memories with emotion from the mood would therefore provide them with a *selective localization advantage* not shared by memories without these specific emotional associations. The final combination of matched memories would be those that most closely corresponded to the array of emotional and nonemotional associations present. Such memories would enter consciousness as the interpretation for the original perception.

Assume that the final combination of matched memories corresponding to the original perception was associated with emotions A, E, and F. In this case, only emotion A from the original mood would have contributed to the final selection of matched memories. We can assume that those stored memories linked to emotions B, C, and D did not receive enough support from nonemotional associations of the incoming perception for full activation. Such memories would therefore not have become part of the final interpretation. Emotions A, E, and F would be released from the activated memories and enter the mood to complement the original four.

INTENSITY OF EMOTION IN THE MOOD

Presumably the intensity of emotion present in the mood decreases over time if it is not periodically reinforced. This is based on the general observation that moods seem to gradually fade without constant stimulation. In the previous example, emotion A would be strengthened through the matching process, while B, C, and D would continue to decay at some natural rate. New interpretations thus serve to alter the prevailing mood by adding new components and strengthening those emotions that are common. In this way, the composition of the mood and the intensities of its components may change over time as memories and new thoughts pass through consciousness.

In this example, emotion A was in association with the complex of memories activated in the localization process. As explained earlier, one or more of the memories that arose during the interpretation process may have been the original contributor of this emotion to the mood. In this way, a recent thought or memory may play a role in a current interpretation. Had more of the original emotions from the mood been matched, perhaps a higher percentage of recent thoughts or memories would have been included in the final interpretation. In this way, emotions composing the mood may provide a reference to recent mental activity, thus maintaining the current relevance and focus of thought.

MOOD AS A BLENDING OF EMOTION

As suggested here, mood may be viewed as a blending of emotions sensed cumulatively in consciousness. Presumably, the ongoing process of interpretation would yield emotions of many different intensities and types. The overall emotional tone present should therefore be a general measure of these variables. For example, a strong negative emotion may almost completely outweigh one or more weaker positive emotions. This would seem to be a consequence of the blended nature of emotions composing the mood. In addition, older emotions present in the mood would be expected to be weaker that those of equal initial strength added at a later time. Because of natural decay, we can predict that in most cases an emotional interpretation from a recent thought would be more dominant in the mood than emotions added earlier. For this reason, emotion derived from any current interpretation should stand out in the mood, allowing it to be distinguished from those that have faded somewhat. Obviously a number of factors may determine which emotions would dominate the emotional state at any given time.

MEMORY RECALL IS MOOD-SPECIFIC

In this chapter, an explanation of the effects observed in state-dependency has been presented. It is postulated that the principles underlying this process may be widespread and influence all thinking. By assuming that memory recall is mood-specific, the apparent ability of emotion to guide and direct thought can be understood. The principles of state-dependency may also help to explain various forms of organic as well as functional amnesia. This will be discussed in the next chapter.

Amnesia and Dissociative Phenomena

As postulated earlier, memory retrieval may be a function of the existing mood. The dominant emotional state present at any time may selectively determine the availability of memories that can be retrieved. If an incompatibility existed between the emotional elements of a current mood and those associated with a memory in storage, the ability to localize and recall such an entity during thought might be reduced. Occasionally such an emotional mismatch may be so great that memory retrieval would fail completely. Amnesia for emotionally incompatible memories would exist as long as the mood state prevailed and external perception did not provide a sufficient number of nonemotional cues to produce localization. Retrieval of such memories would only become feasible once a more emotionally harmonious mood was generated. These ideas seem to underlie the phenomenon of state-dependency and may also explain how emotion guides thought. Could this hypothesis also explain the selective amnesia characteristic of multiple personality disorder (MPD) and other dissociative phenomena? These fascinating possibilities will be examined.

MULTIPLE PERSONALITY DISORDER

MPD is a relatively rare condition that is seen most often in women exposed to emotional trauma early in life (Putnam, Guroff, Silberman, Barban, & Post, 1986; Ross, Norton, & Wozney, 1989). Individuals with this disorder often seem to possess two or more separate personality structures, which are expressed at different times. Each personality appears to be self-contained and independent of the others (Bliss, 1980). In some cases, individual personalities may be so isolated that each is totally unaware of the others. In many cases the lines of separation may not be so clear, and each may possess some knowledge of the others. Occasionally, one or more personalities may have full knowledge of another, but there may be no reciprocal awareness. Considerable variation in amnestic patterns may exist from one case to the next. Such personalities may be radically different in attitudes toward life, morals, expressions of emotion, speech patterns, and even handwriting. It has even been claimed that vital signs and other physical parameters may differ from one entity to the next. This fascinating disorder is reviewed in recent books by Putnam (1989) and Ross (1989).

MPD is classified as a dissociative phenomenon because of the apparent fragmentation it produces in personality structure. In many cases, a part of self appears to *split off* and take on its own separate identity. In the great majority of cases seen in modern psychiatry, MPD seems to result from early childhood emotional or physical trauma (Putnam et al., 1986; Ross et al., 1989). This usually involves sexual abuse but can arise from any type of prolonged trauma. It is frequently difficult to recognize and may initially present as a mixture of depression, anxiety, nightmares, bizarre behavior, mood swings, and emotional liability. There may be no initial complaint of early emotional trauma. These people are often misdiagnosed as suffering from an affective disorder, schizophrenia, or are felt to have a severe personality disorder (Ross et al., 1989). Failure of such patients to respond to conventional treatment may be a clue that the diagnosis is in error (Kluft, 1985).

Frequently, the patient may indicate that she has trouble with time. Closer questioning may reveal that the patient may have frequent amnestic episodes, lasting from hours to days. In effect, she may report that there is a loss of time in her life for which she can not account. Others may tell her of things she did or said, for which she has no memory. The patient may have experienced these lapses in memory for years and view them as normal. Such amnestic episodes are generally felt to be shifts into alternate personality states, which are amnestic to the primary personality. This is frequently the main clue to MPD for the examining psychiatrist.

PREVIOUS THEORIES OF MULTIPLE PERSONALITY DISORDER

Many theories have been proposed through the years to explain MPD (Andorfer, 1985; Bliss, 1986; Brende, 1984; Kluft, 1984, Spanos, Weekes, &

Bertrand, 1985). The hypothesis presented in this work suggests that state-dependent memory effects may partially underlie the phenomena of MPD. This is consistent with some earlier theories of MPD, which used state-dependent learning effects to explain the amnesia seen in this disorder (Braun, 1984; Kluft, 1984; Ludwig, Brandsma, Wilber, Bendfeldt, & Jameson, 1972; Putnam, 1986; Ribot, 1910). As indicated in the following hypothesis, a number of factors may be involved in its etiology and maintenance.

EVOLUTION OF MULTIPLE PERSONALITY DISORDER

We can speculate that the process of MPD begins when a severe emotional trauma experienced by a child generates a unique combination of emotions that become part of the existing mood. Because of the relative inexperience of the child, such emotions and events may not have been encountered previously. These entities would therefore have no prior association from direct experience. This, of course, would not be surprising in a young child. For an emotional understanding of the situation to occur, it would be compared with the child's store of inherited, generalized knowledge. The matching of corresponding data would produce the activation of appropriate emotions that would enter the mood to provide interpretation. Such emotions would therefore acquire their first associated memories from direct experience as a result of the abusive conditions. On each subsequent episode of trauma, new memories would become associated with this specific mood state. In this way, an entire complex of related memories may accumulate and become specifically associated with one unique combination of emotions experienced only during abusive episodes. Such events may generate the conditions of memory isolation that are probably necessary for the development of MPD.

The theory of state-dependency proposed here suggests that memories associate with specific emotions that serve as retrieval cues in the localization process. Such entities function along with other associations to provide each memory with a specific and separate identity. The recall of memories originally stored in one emotional context may therefore be facilitated in the presence of the same mood state. Under these conditions, the emotional cues required for localization would be present in the prevailing mood. This process was discussed earlier. Presumably, retrieval becomes increasingly more difficult as the composition of the mood moves away from the original emotional state existing at the time of storage. In the presence of very different moods, memory recall may be virtually impossible. This is presumably a rare situation, because most memories are probably associated with a variety of common emotions that would correspond, at least in part, to most moods and promote some recall. The generation of a mood totally incompatible with some degree of memory retrieval would be unusual. In other words, most moods probably support some recall of most memories.

The *unique mood state* generated during abusive episodes would be indicative of an unusual or rare, traumatic situation. The emotional components associated with such memories would presumably be very intense and strong because of the frightening nature of the trauma, and would exclusively reflect the original abusive experiences. As discussed before, such emotional associations would function as important cues in any subsequent retrieval of this information into consciousness. In the absence of such emotional data in an existing mood, memory recall would be difficult or impossible unless the original situation itself were repeated.

INITIAL ASSOCIATION OF MEMORY WITH EMOTION

The initial association of memories with inherited emotion, as described here, is probably a *normal occurrence*, which is by no means unique to MPD. From ideas presented earlier, it would be expected that every *primal emotion* existing in an infant would eventually combine with a memory in its first associative relationship. This is probably an active process in early childhood when new experiences happen almost daily. When this first occurs, an exclusive association should be established between the elements involved. Over time, we can speculate that a *blending process* would occur, allowing integration of these memories and emotions with others similar entities. In effect, further associative relationships would develop through new experience, which would end the original exclusive pairing. If this did not occur, memories and their emotional components would remain in virtual isolation from each other. Under these conditions, the extensive associative connections necessary for memory localization and recall would not develop. The hypothesis presented here predicts several ways this normal blending process might be achieved. This will be briefly discussed.

BLENDING OF MEMORY WITH EMOTION

Blending may occur when unrelated events stimulate the same basic emotions to enter the mood. For example, many things with no apparent connection may make us laugh, stimulate anger, or induce anxiety. In this way, a number of dissimilar events may eventually link with a single emotion or a specific combination of such entities, providing them with an associated relationship in memory. Over time, it is conceivable that primal emotions might come to share many memories through this process. In other words, memories of numerous events from experience may eventually link with one or more primal emotions, which would provide them with associative blending. A mood containing such an emotion would favor the recall of all those memories to which it had become linked. From this grouping of memories, any nonemotional cues present would further specify the particular memory that was ultimately brought into consciousness. Memories would thus become integrated with each other through the sharing of common emotions. Although a number of other mechanisms for blending might be postulated, this will be the only one discussed at this time.

In the *blending process* described, memories and emotions are considered to be physically related through association. As a consequence, structures encoding emotional information are activated when memories are used in cognition. Others have postulated similar systems of neural organization. In the differential emotions theory proposed by Izard (1977), functionally analogous neural complexes are referred to as affective–cognitive structures. Tomkins's (1962, 1963) *ideoaffective organization* is also similar to this blending process.

FAILURE OF BLENDING IN MULTIPLE PERSONALITY DISORDER

In childhood abuse, the normal blending process described may not occur to any significant extent. The traumatic experience might generate a *unique emotional response* not easily reproducible by other events in life. Under these conditions, the emotions involved would not acquire memories of things separate from the abusive episodes. The conditions necessary for the generation of this specific mood state would simply be too rare. In effect, such memories would not blend extensively with other memories acquired by the brain. A single complex of memories tied to a specific emotional pattern would accumulate in *virtual isolation*. This should greatly restrict the conditions under which such memories could be recalled, and would produce the conditions necessary for the development of MPD. This is illustrated in Figure 7.1.

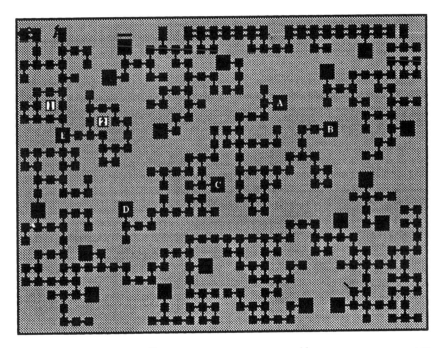

Figure 7.1 In this figure, small squares represent neurons, and larger squares represent associated emotion. Memories that support an alternate personality structure are shown isolated in the center of this figure and are associated with emotions *A–D*. Note that there are no synaptic linkages connecting this grouping of memories with the main body of stored entities, which contains the primary personality. Note that emotion *E* connects memories 1 and 2 to the main body of memories and thus represents a form of "emotional blending," which is explained in the text.

RECALL OF TRAUMATIC MEMORIES

For memories of the abusive situation to be recalled, elements of the original unique mood would need to be present to facilitate the localization process. But generation of such a mood would occur *only when a situation similar to the original was experienced*. It seems unlikely that reestablishment of such a mood could be accomplished during routine thinking or nonabusive circumstances. As indicated, there would be little if any blending of normal memories with those of the original abuse. *In effect, there would be no associative routes leading to such memories.* This should effectively prevent the recall of traumatic memories or the corresponding mood in normal thought. During *nonabusive* times, there would essentially be *no awareness for such events, because nothing would be present to re-*

generate the original mood state. This would depend exclusively upon a recurrence of events similar to the original trauma. Such a situation would greatly limit the conditions under which memories of the trauma could be brought into consciousness.

During an episode of abuse, a mood state compatible with recall of prior traumatic memories would be generated. After the episode ended and the thoughts of the abuse passed from consciousness, the specific mood elements necessary for recall would no longer continue to be actively generated. The mood would change to reflect the current situation. In the absence of this specific mood state, recall of the same traumatic memories would no longer be possible, because the emotional cues necessary for retrieval would be absent. At this point, the brain would probably have little awareness of such memories. *The only way these entities could be called back into consciousness would be a repeat of the original abusive situation. If this occurred, enough retrieval cues would presumably be present for localization of the involved memories without the need for emotional information*. The events of the new episode would restore the original mood, and recall of all memories linked to this specific set of emotions would again be possible. When the episode ended, the mood would again fade, and the brain would become amnestic for the memories of the trauma.

As suggested, the mood generated by an abusive situation would need to be free of prior association for the isolated conditions necessary for MPD to develop. Too better understand this concept, let us assume that such a mood state had prior associations acquired from experience. In such a case, many situations and thoughts *other than those surrounding the abuse itself* might trigger a mood compatible with recall of the abusive memories. If nonemotional cues peripherally related to the abuse were also available, memories of the original situation might be specified and recalled. A repeat of the original abusive episode would *not be necessary* for the events of the trauma to be remembered. It is obvious that such traumatic memories would not remain isolated under these conditions, and MPD would not develop. Under these conditions, many related thoughts and events might indirectly produce recall. Numerous routes might thus be available by which these traumatic memories could be brought into consciousness.

ALTERNATE PERSONALITIES

In the case of *repeating trauma* such as sexual abuse, various adaptive coping styles may develop. Over time, the individual may develop new strategies that ease the pain of the situation. This may involve different ways of interacting or dealing with the sexual perpetrator. For example, a child may learn that certain attitudes or actions provide more protection than others. In effect, he or she may learn to cope through experience. Over an extended time, many characteristics of personality may become involved that specifically associate with the unique mood state present during the abuse. Such new personality traits would, of course, be manifest only during times of abuse because of their exclusive association with the traumatic mood. At other times, this complex of new personality characteristics would not be retrievable because of an incompatibly with the normal mood. They would effectively remain isolated from the original personality structure. This would be the origin of the *alternate personalities* that develop in MPD.

DEVELOPING NEW COPING STYLES

Developing new coping styles in response to stressful or challenging situations is certainly not unique to victims of childhood abuse. This occurs in all of us as a natural consequence of any new situation we experience. New personality traits may develop in any child subjected to an altered set of circumstances over time. This is part of the normal process of learning and growing. In MPD, the unique mood state may prevent these new characteristics from being integrated into the normal structure of the personality. In effect, there would be a segregation of personality characteristics, which develop because of the selective memory recall provided by the traumatic mood. In the absence of conditions leading to MPD, such new adaptive traits would be perceived only as subtle changes in the normal personality structure of the child. No separate entity would develop under these conditions.

SELECTIVE AWARENESS

If the abusive situation continued over an extended period, the state of isolation imposed by the mood might not remain complete. Some *blending* of memories or emotions between the normal and traumatic mood states might conceivably occur. Through this process, the various personalities might gain some awareness of each other. It is certainly possible that the blending process might not be equal in all directions. This might produce a type of *selective awareness* in some personalities but not in others. Some entities may thus have a more complete level of knowledge of their mental environment than others. Many patterns of amnesia might thus be established, depending upon the specific situations involved.

GENERALIZATION OF STIMULUS ELEMENTS

The low level of blending postulated to occur over time between isolated mood states may have another important consequence. Such changes should permit conditions *other than those identical to the initial trauma* to induce the unique mood state. In effect, some generalization of the original stimulus conditions might eventually develop, allowing the emergence of an alternate personality in more general situations. *Under these conditions, an alternate personality structure might appear in response to a number of frightening events other than those that produced the original trauma. If some degree of stimulus generalization did not occur, altered personality states could not be observed in conditions other than those that originally produced them.* Thus, some blending of mood states seems necessary for the full expression of MPD.

DURATION OF ABUSE

The development of one or more alternate personalities may be a function of the *duration* of the abuse experienced. The adaptive changes that probably form the basis for new personality structures may only occur when abuse is repetitive and continued over a prolonged period of time. A single traumatic episode or a brief sequence of such events may not provide an adequate opportunity for adaptive changes to be implemented. MPD would therefore not have the chance to fully develop.

ABUSE OF A SHORTER DURATION

The mood state unique to an abusive situation would, however, still be generated when the abuse was of shorter duration. Even though no alternate personality may develop, there should still be amnesia for the traumatic events, for the reasons described earlier. This is actually very common in victims of childhood abuse who do not develop MPD. Often there will be no apparent knowledge of the abusive events for many years. Such early trauma may have no obvious effect on the patient's life. In their 20s or 30s, such individuals often report the sudden onset of

bothersome nightmares or flashback memories, which they do not understand. Over time, memory fragments or whole memories may return.
Slowly, the full picture of childhood abuse may emerge and become apparent to the patient. This is often so emotionally devastating that hospitalization and long-term psychotherapy, combined with medication,
may be necessary.

REPRESSION

The inability to recall memories of childhood trauma is usually attributed to *repression*. This classic, psychological process is considered to be
involuntary and was originally described by Sigmund Freud many
years ago. Repression is usually viewed as the most important way the
brain protects itself from the painful and unpleasant memories it stores.
For this reason, it is referred to as a *defense mechanism*. The ideas presented here seem to provide a basis for the mechanism by which memories of childhood abuse are hidden from conscious view.

FAILURE OF MULTIPLE PERSONALITY DISORDER
TO DEVELOP IN ADULTS

MPD is a phenomenon that seems to arise *exclusively from early childhood
trauma*. Adults who experience comparable emotional distress do not
seem to develop this syndrome and usually experience no amnesia for
the traumatic events. The conditions responsible for the generation of
MPD obviously do not fully exist in adults. As indicated earlier, the
emotions used to generate the unique mood state accompanying childhood abuse may have no prior use in experience. Their incorporation
into the traumatic mood may be their first chance to enter association
with memory. This probably forms the basis for the separation of different personality structures that has been observed in MPD. *In adults, most
primary emotions or combinations of emotions probably have some prior usage.*
In other words, most common emotions probably exist in association
with memory to one extent or another. There would be few unique emotions, alone or in combination, still existing. The emotions generated as a
result of a severe trauma suffered by an adult would in most cases have
some prior reference in experience. The memories of trauma experienced by an adult would therefore not be stored in isolation. Such memories could be triggered by cues other than those of the traumatic event
itself. Many access routes might thus be available to these memories if

the involved emotions had a reasonable degree of prior usage. The specific conditions necessary for the development of isolated memories would therefore not exist, and MPD would not arise.

EVOLUTION OF MORE THAN ONE ALTERNATE PERSONALITY

The generation of more than one alternate personality state may reflect *a change in the basic pattern of abuse.* In other words, a second form of related trauma may arise, or the original episodes may change in such a way as to necessitate new adaptive styles. Every significant change in the abusive situation may alter the traumatic emotional pattern slightly, providing each new alternate with *its own specific mood.* In effect, the original process described may be duplicated, at least in part, for each new entity that emerges.

In a sense, MPD may be viewed as a failure to adequately mix mental entities in a normal way. Presumably, all early memories linked to primal emotion would initially experience some degree of isolation. Such memories would eventually become integrated into the overall mental perspective as the primal emotion acquired other associations. In rare cases, the emotional composition of the mood generated might be so unique that this normal blending process would fail, and an isolated pocket of memory would result. An adaptive personality style, indicative of the situation, may evolve in this isolated domain and be viewed as a separate personality.

BORDERLINE PERSONALITY DISORDER

It is unlikely that the development of MPD is an *all or nothing* phenomenon. Many variations of MPD may be possible, reflecting different degrees of memory integration. In a few cases, little memory blending may be present, and classic MPD may be observed. In perhaps many more cases, higher degrees of integration may have occurred, producing a less well-defined clinical picture. A sufficient degree of memory integration may be present, so that overt amnesia is not produced. Even so, enough memory isolation may have originally occurred to allow some adaptive personality traits to associate with each separate emotional state encountered. Under these conditions, changes in mood status might bring about dramatic alterations in thought content and behavior, but without the complete switch in personality structure seen in full-blown MPD. In effect, a milder form of MPD may exist, which is much less recognizable than the full syndrome.

Such patients may seem to live in a chaotic world. Their emotional reactions to trivial events may seem grossly out of proportion. They may repeatedly form intense interpersonal relationships that fragment at the slightest provocation. Extremes in behavior may be commonplace as mood changes allow different adaptive personality traits to emerge. Events in life may be viewed as all *black or white*. In other words, subtle differences in situations may be difficult to realize because of the strong emotional bias imposed by a poorly integrated mood state. Things may thus be viewed as all good or bad with no middle ground. In psychological terms, this is known as *splitting*.

Under conditions of stress, such personality structures may seem to become disorganized and perhaps fragmented. The individual may seem to display brief periods of psychosis because of the erratic and perhaps frequent changes observed in personality. Such patients may possess many poorly integrated personality traits that are extremely mood specific. In effect, this chaotic form of personality structure may represent a variation of MPD. This condition is probably synonymous with *borderline personality disorder* (BPD). This is a well-characterized and severely pathological form of personality structure that is known to share many common elements with MPD. Like MPD, BPD is frequently associated with severe childhood trauma. In addition, MPD patients who have been tested with the Minnesota Multiphasic Personality Inventory often show profiles that are commonly regarded as indicative of BPD (Bliss, 1984; Coons & Sterne, 1986; Solomon, 1983). This popular psychological test has been widely administered to patients with MPD.

A CONTINUUM OF MOOD INTEGRATION

In the *normal* personality structure, integration of mood states may be more complete, although probably not total. Some separation presumably exists, allowing us to utilize selective memory recall to advantage. As indicated before, the bias imposed by various emotional states may guide and direct thought to reflect current concerns. Without some degree of emotional isolation, thinking might be more random and less well directed. A *continuum of mood integration* may exist, with MPD at one extreme and normal personality at the other. BPD would occupy some intermediate position.

The affective instability that seems to characterize BPD has led some researchers to suggest that it may actually represent a subsyndromal type of mood disorder (Akiskal, Yerevanian, Davis, King, & Lemmi, 1985; Gunderson & Elliott, 1985), whereas others (McGlashan, 1983; Pope, Jonas, Hudson, Cohen, & Gunderson, 1983) maintain that it is a true disorder of personality that frequently coexists with affective disorder. *The theoretical concepts presented here suggest that BPD may actually be a form of dissociative disorder.* Others have arrived at the same conclusion, based upon the general characteristics of this disorder (Ross, 1989).

HALLUCINATIONS IN MULTIPLE PERSONALITY DISORDER

According to those who have studied MPD extensively, *auditory hallucinations* in this disorder are a frequent occurrence (Bliss, Larson, & Nakashima, 1983, Putnam et al., 1986). In fact, the majority of MPD patients experience this type of hallucination, but most are reluctant to admit this early in therapy. These voices are generally clear and distinct, and are usually experienced by the host (original or primary) personality. They may provide a running commentary on various aspects of the patient's life and often seem completely realistic and coherent. Occasionally they criticize or belittle the patient and may command him or her to commit suicide or to engage in a wide assortment of harmful acts. In some cases, more than one voice may be present. Therapists who are familiar with MPD generally feel that these voices originate from alternate personality states. In some way, verbal thoughts arising from one or more personalities seem to be perceived by the host. They are often frightening for the primary personality, who may have no understanding of their origin.

THEORETICAL EXPLANATION FOR AUDITORY HALLUCINATIONS

The hypothesis proposed suggests that the host personality, in most cases, is amnestic for memories acquired by an alternate personality. As explained earlier, such memories are tied to emotion that is in the exclusive domain of the alternate state. In the absence of such emotions in the current mood, the host personality would be unable to localize and retrieve these memories. For this reason, memories linked with an alternate personality would not normally be recalled by the host personality during routine thought. The only way such entities could be accessed would be for events *very similar* to those that produced the original memories to be experienced again. Under these conditions, localization *would not require* compatible emotion to be present in the host mood. The preponderance of nonemotional cues, generated by the situation, should *alone* be sufficient to support localization. In such cases, localized memories associated with the alternate state would be activated and their associated emotion released into the mood as an interpretation. If this emotion was of *significant intensity,* a mood characteristic of the alternate state should fully emerge in consciousness, allowing those memories associated with this domain to become readily available for recall. Although the process of "switching" from one personality to another seems mysterious and complicated, *it may simply be viewed as a change in the emotional composition of a dominate mood to one that supports the recall of a different grouping of memories.* As indicated earlier, this may be the mechanism by which switching between "personalities" occurs in MPD.

From the previous scenario, a *rational explanation* for auditory hallucinations can be postulated. Because moods appear to be a combination of many emotions that are sensed cumulatively in consciousness, a significant amount of emotional release may be necessary to produce a complete switch or change from a mood supporting one personality state to another. In some cases, the emotion that emerges from interpretations arising from a nondominant, alternate personality store of memories *may not be of sufficient intensity* to overcome or completely replace the prevailing host mood. Such new emotion may alter the existing emotional tone *but not enough to supplant it as the dominant entity in consciousness.* The existing mood should still be capable of supporting the host personality state in such cases. Under these conditions, verbal interpretations, arising from an alternate personality's storage of memories, would appear alien to the host personality still in consciousness. This mood state would simply *not provide access* to those memories necessary for the understanding and interpretation of these entities. Such verbal thoughts would therefore appear strange and *not of self* to the host personality, and would be viewed as auditory hallucinations by an examining psychiatrist.

It is therefore proposed that auditory hallucinations in MPD occur when interpretive emotion from an alternate state, which *does not have the intensity to produce a full switch in mood content,* enters consciousness. Under such conditions, the host state would remain dominate but be unable to interpret thoughts and words arising from alternate personality structures. When such *alien* emotion eventually faded from the mood, localization of memories from the alternate grouping of memories would no longer be supported, and the *voices* would disappear from consciousness. Alternately, if sufficient alter emotion accumulated in consciousness through ongoing interpretation, the mood should become dominated by such emotion, and a *full switch* to a secondary state should occur. Verbal thought, arising from this personality structure, would now be recognized as familiar to the alter entity occupying consciousness. Of course, any thought that arose and entered consciousness at this point from the host personality structure might be viewed as alien to the dominate alter state.

The mechanism proposed here for the generation of auditory hallucinations in MPD is probably different from that occurring in primary psychotic disorders. This assumption is based upon the observation that the brains of schizophrenic patients show gross organic changes, which are not seen in MPD or mood disorders. In addition, auditory hallucinations in MPD are largely perceived as alien thoughts or voices arising from *within the head*, whereas those occurring in schizophrenia often seem to enter the ears from *external sources*. There may also be a differential response to antipsychotic medications in these two patient groups. It is my personal observation that the auditory hallucinations of MPD are much less responsive to this type of treatment than those arising in schizophrenia. As will be explained in a later chapter, the auditory hallucinations that often accompany depression and mania probably arise in *exactly the same way* as proposed for MPD and may therefore utilize the same mechanism.

SIMULTANEOUS CYCLES OF THOUGHT

The ideas proposed here suggest that two simultaneous cycles of thought may exist under conditions that foster hallucinations. One would originate from the host and the other from the alternate state. Both cycles would be initiated from a single event *simultaneously processed* by each personality structure. Under these conditions, each state would produce an independent interpretation based upon its own individual store of memories. Both sets of interpretations would be sensed in consciousness by the host personality. The one arising from the alternate state would not be recognizable by the host personality, and would be perceived as an alien voice. This might be followed by additional interpretive rounds in each personality domain, resulting in a continuation of both cycles. Under such conditions, only the host personality would experience active awareness of the cycling thoughts, because it would dominate the prevailing mood. If awareness existed in the alternate state, it would not be sensed at a conscious level.

PSYCHOGENIC AMNESIA

The hypothesis presented here may also help to explain psychogenic amnesia. This is considered to be a rare dissociative state arising exclusively from emotional trauma. Accounts of this fascinating phenomenon are occasionally reported by the news media. Typical situations often involve individuals who have lost all memory of past life. They may be found wandering aimlessly and be unable to remember their name, address, or any details of their personal circumstances (Rapaport, 1971). Despite this, they may retain the ability to drive a car, to dress themselves, and perform many routine daily tasks necessary for normal living. In effect, their memory loss appears to be highly selective. The amnestic state typically lasts from hours to days, but rare cases may continue for years. *When recovery finally occurs and memories are restored, there is often an inability to recall the events of the amnestic period itself. One set of memories seems to be exchanged for another.*

The events precipitating this form of amnesia may not differ significantly from those leading to MPD. Traumatic life events may generate a highly unique emotional state not previously encountered by the individual. Presumably, some rare combination of emotions may remain free of associations, even into adulthood, in some individuals. Deeply disturbing and completely new experiences might conceivably trigger such a mood state. This is probably a rare occurrence in the general population and may explain the extremely low incidence of psychogenic amnesia. Such a mood state might be totally incompatible with memories of prior life events. Under these conditions, the individual may experience a total inability to retrieve past memories that require emotional association for localization. Amnesia would continue until circumstances created a change in mood.

In contrast to memories that are forgotten, there seems to be a selective retention for certain types of knowledge in psychogenic amnesia. As indicated earlier, individuals with this disorder may retain the ability to perform many routine daily tasks and utilize language. Perhaps such memories do not require emotional cues for localization. It is conceivable that some heavily used memories may lose this form of associative identification through a process of *emotional dilution*, which will be described fully in the next chapter. It may also be possible that many procedural-type memories may not require associated emotion for retrieval. This is further discussed in the section on amnesia resulting from hippocampal loss. *Regardless of the exact cause, such memories probably remain available, because they do not rely on emotions as retrieval cues.* This may explain the selective pattern of amnesia often observed in this disorder.

Memories stored during an amnestic period are often not remembered once the episode clears. This observation is also consistent with the idea that selective recall is a function of mood state. In other words, the restored mood might not support retrieval of memories accumulated during the emotional state of the amnestic episode. *One amnestic state might thus be swapped for another when the dominant mood changes.*

THE HIPPOCAMPUS AND MEMORY STORAGE

The work presented here would not be complete without some mention of the *hippocampus* and its relationship to memory storage. There is an extensive literature on this subject, for which reviews are currently available (Eichenbaum, Otto, & Cohen, 1992; Squire, 1992). The two lobes of this brain structure are located bilaterally on the medial aspect of each temporal lobe and are considered to be a part of the limbic system. The hippocampus is thought to be extensively connected to most, if not all, sensory systems of the cortex (Squire & Zola-Morgan, 1988). The bilateral resection of this structure in humans is known to produce anterograde amnesia (*medial-temporal-lobe amnesia*), as in the well-publicized case of patient H. M. (Milner, 1970; Milner, Corkin, & Teuber, 1968; Scoville & Milner, 1957). Patients with bilateral loss or extensive damage of this structure are unable to convert short-term memory into more permanent forms. Events may be retained within the brain for a few minutes but are totally lost once short-term memory decays. Interestingly, these patients can still recall and utilize memories stored before hippocampal loss. This structure, therefore, seems to have little if any detectable bearing on these processes. *The functional defect seems to be an inability to incorporate or consolidate new learning.*

MEDIAL-TEMPORAL-LOBE AMNESIA

Although the type of amnesia exhibited by H. M. is usually attributed to hippocampal loss, bilateral-medial temporal lobectomy actually produces damage to several major brain structures. Because of this, three competing neuroanatomical hypotheses have arisen to explain medial-temporal-lobe amnesia.

The first is that of Scoville and Milner (1957) which suggests that hippocampal damage is the main event precipitating this syndrome. In 1978, Mishkin proposed that both hippocampal and amygdaloid injury are necessary for this type of amnesia to develop. The final hypothesis, proposed by Horel in 1978, suggests that the temporal stem, which is adjacent to the hippocampus and amygdala, is the actual structure involved. Although this issue still remains unresolved, in this work, damage to the hippocampus will be considered to be the chief cause of medial-temporal-lobe amnesia although the amygdala may certainly be involved. Research with animals has indicated that the amygdala may be central to the acquisition and expression of new learning associated with fear (Davis, 1992; Gray, 1989; Kapp & Pascoe, 1986; Kapp, Pascoe, & Bixler, 1984). The role of the amygdala in learning is discussed later in this chapter.

THE HIPPOCAMPUS AND CONDITIONED LEARNING

In studies involving *conditioned learning,* an increase in the rate of firing was observed in pyramidal cells in the dorsal hippocampus, even before a conditioned response could be detected (Berger & Thompson, 1978a, 1978b). This structure therefore seems to be participating in the storage of new memories. Various interfering manipulations such as electroconvulsive shock (Duncan, 1949) or head trauma (Russell & Nathan, 1946) are known to disrupt memory storage if done shortly after a learning experience. These type experiments have generally been interpreted as evidence that new memories must undergo a process of consolidation or maturation after they are initially registered in the brain. It has been suggested that this may be mediated by the hippocampus and perhaps the neighboring amygdala.

THE HIPPOCAMPUS AS A REPEATING CIRCUIT

It seems possible that the hippocampus serves as a *repeating circuit,* causing the repetitive firing of memories undergoing consolidation at a locus outside the hippocampus. It can be assumed that storage of long-term memory occurs outside of the hippocampus in humans, because damage to this structure does not cause major retrograde amnesia (Squire, 1986, 1987b). Following initial activation of the primitive memory, the energy discharged might be channeled to the hippocampus and reflected back on the new structure. This would result in a second activation, and the process would be repeated. On each cycle, the hippocampus may provide amplifying energy, enabling the process to continue. In effect, there would be a repetitive activation of the new memory, driven by the hippocampus in cyclic fashion. This would continue until the new memory structure was sufficiently consolidated. Presumably, this would involve a strengthening of synaptic linkages or an increase in their absolute number, thus electrically linking the pieces of the new memory into a coherent structure. These ideas are anatomically feasible, because the hippocampus is known to have an extensive system of feedback fibers, which link it back to its original source of input from the neocortex (Van Hoesen, 1982). In effect, the hippocampus can theoretically influence the neocortical areas from which it receives inputs through these feedback circuits. These ideas are similar in many ways to those presented by Mishkin and Appenzeller (1987) and others (e.g., Rolls, 1990).

EMOTIONAL INTENSITY MAY DRIVE HIPPOCAMPAL ACTIVITY

The hypothesis presented here suggests that the process described might be driven by the *emotion* associated with the new memory. The *intensity* of this associated component may determine the number of

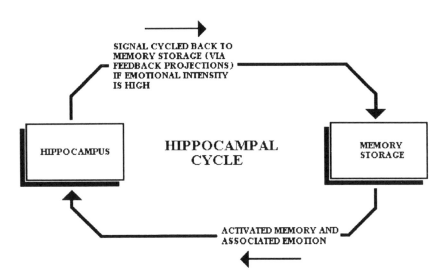

Figure 7.2 It is proposed that the hippocampus stimulates memory consolidation by repeatedly activating structures that are associated with strong emotion. In this way, important memories, which are generally associated with significant levels of emotion, become reinforced so they are preserved for future reference. This cyclic mechanism is illustrated here. Through the process of *emotional dilution* (defined and discussed in Chapter 8), associated emotion dissipates until the cycle slows and eventually ends.

reinforcing cycles and therefore the final strength of the memory. This is consistent with the observation that memories stored during intense emotion are usually very strong and durable. It is also in agreement with the work of Berger and Thompson (1987a, 1987b) who observed that the firing rates of hippocampal cells seemed to parallel the strength of conditioning. In their experiments, Pavlovian conditioning of the nictitating membranes of rabbits was accomplished using a tone as the conditioned stimulus and an air puff as the unconditioned stimulus. The animals were strapped down during these experiments to prevent movement from interfering with the electrical recording. This appears to be a standard procedure in work of this type. Under such conditions, it seems likely that most animals would experience a considerable amount of fear, apprehension, and anxiety. In effect, such experimental conditions may have generated emotion that influenced the final outcome. Perhaps the *emotional response* to these conditions was the *actual driving force* for hippocampal activity, which was observed during the course of learning. As a part of the limbic system, the hippocampus would seem ideally suited to drive emotional learning. These ideas are illustrated in Figure 7.2.

REPETITION IN MEMORY STORAGE

An event that yields a strong emotional interpretation *may not need to be experienced more than once to produce a durable memory*. The intense emotion released during the evaluation of such incoming data may drive the hippocampus until the new structure is strongly reinforced. Events with a low degree of emotional association may not be stored so easily. In addition to a small emotional drive from the hippocampus, their consolidation may require repetition from experience to become strongly fixed. *In other words, the repetition necessary to acquire such a memory may come from experience as well as hippocampal drive.* An arrangement such as this would allow memories to be stored according to their *relative importance* to the brain or their *usage in experience*. Memories of most routine daily activities would be weakly stored, whereas those few events that occur with some frequency, or have significant emotional connotation, would be more strongly reinforced. These ideas suggest that the process of consolidation might go on for perhaps years, if experience continued to provide repetition, or if recall of the memory produced sustained emotion. The strength or retention of such a memory might subsequently decline once its relevance to current life events passed. This is consistent with the general proposition presented in this work that memories are not static, but undergo continual remodeling to reflect their prevailing usage. The idea that consolidation may continue to occur *over a significant portion of the lifetime of the memory* was suggested by Squire in 1986.

REPETITION IN THE CONSOLIDATION PROCESS

The hypothesis presented here predicts that all new data entering the brain would acquire some emotional association from the prevailing mood. Such emotion serves as a *contextual environment*, which frames all our thoughts and activities. Every new memory would therefore receive some emotional drive from the hippocampus as a result of this form of association. Because intensity of the mood can vary greatly, hippocampal reinforcement might produce very weak transient memories or those that are very strong and lasting. Thus, the ultimate strength of a memory would seem to result from a combination of repetition it received through experience over time and whatever drive it received from the hippocampus. Repetition is proposed here to be the single common factor necessary for memory reinforcement in the consolidation process.

TYPES OF LONG-TERM MEMORY

The memory deficits seen in amnestic patients can usually be described as disruptions in one or more of the three types of long-term memories thought to exist. These forms include *episodic, semantic,* and *procedural memory* (Tulving, 1983, 1985). In some literature, episodic and semantic memories may be referred to as *declarative memory*. The most consistently affected form of memory in anterograde amnesia is episodic. Patients are generally unable to remember the events in their lives for over 1 minute. In effect, the episodes that constitute their daily activities and experiences cannot be converted into long-term form. Semantic memory is also severely disrupted in most cases. New words and their definitions, or lists of words, which are studied for future recall, are usually not retained. In a few cases, however, some ability to acquire new semantic information may remain. For example, some verbally learned facts are apparently stored and can be recalled later but surprisingly, individuals are usually unable to remember where or when they learned this new information. This interesting phenomenon seems to represent a dissociation between semantic and episodic memories, and has been termed *source amnesia* (Schacter, Harbluk, & McLachlan, 1984; Shimamura & Squire, 1987).

In contrast to the first two types of memory, which are extensively affected, amnestics usually retain the ability to learn new tasks involving motor skills. Through repetition, these patients can be taught to perform certain tasks involving physical movement. Skill can often be improved with practice. In effect, procedural memory seems to remain largely intact. As with semantic memory, there is usually a dissociation between the memory of the new skill and that of the learning experience itself. Even though patients might be able to perform the motor task, they often cannot remember the events surrounding the learning experience.

EXPLANATION FOR MEMORY DEFICITS IN AMNESIA

Although the memory deficits seen in amnesia are complex, the ideas presented in this work may provide a *theoretical framework for further investigation*. If we apply the concepts presented in this work to the various deficits seen in each type of long-term memory, some understanding of amnesia can be achieved. Let us first consider episodic memory, which is the most severely altered following hippocampal loss. The inability to store this form of memory seems attributable to both an absence of a reinforcing hippocampal drive and a lack of frequently repeating experience. Each new episodic memory we store would normally receive some hippocampal drive, arising from contextual and interpretive emotion. In most cases, this would probably be its main source of reinforcement, because most episodic events may not repeat themselves with any significant frequency. In the absence of a viable hippocampus, no reinforcing energy would reach the new entity, and consolidation would not occur. These structures would receive little repetition from any source and, therefore, would not be stored to any measurable extent. Failure to recall such an entity would simply be due to its *absence* in memory storage.

The deficits seen in semantic memory seem, in some ways, to be similar to those of episodic memory. In fact, this form of memory may actually be just a variation of episodic memory. The two types of memory resemble each other, in that there is often an emotional drive from the hippocampus, which contributes to the consolidation process. Unlike episodic memories, the events that constitute semantic memory may be repeated in experience with some degree of frequency, especially in experimental settings. For example, amnesic patients may be asked to study a list of words so that their retention might be later evaluated. Although there may be no repetition from the hippocampal drive, there is from experience. Unlike episodic memory, the new memory structure would receive some reinforcing energy in this way. Some degree of consolidation would occur under these circumstances, so semantic memory may undergo some consolidation and storage if sufficient repetition from experience occurs.

In most cases, the recall of semantic memories is poor, even when significant experiential repetition is used. In other words, the memory may be present, but it cannot be retrieved. The most likely explanation for this effect is the same phenomenon described for state-dependent memory. Although the memory is present, it lacks an emotional association, which may be critical to retrieval. In other words, the emotional state of the individual during the learning process cannot serve as a retrieval cue. Recall is probably not accomplished, because there is insufficient identifying data to localize and activate the memory in question. With state-dependent memory, recall seems to fail, because testing is attempted in a different emotional state than was present during learning. Under these conditions, the emotion associated with the memory could not serve as a retrieval cue. In semantic memory deficits, no emotion at all is stored, which may produce the same final outcome.

As indicated before, lists of words studied by amnesics are usually poorly recalled. The theory presented here suggests that such words are, in fact, retained in memory but poorly recalled because of retrieval failure. This assumption is supported by the work of Warrington and Weiskrantz (1974). Amnesics who had previously studied a list of words were tested for retention and also given a *stem completion test*. In this test, subjects were shown word stems (words with missing letters) from the original list and asked to fill in the blanks. In normals, retention performance is enhanced if the word stems are derived from words that have recently been presented. This is a form of the *repetition priming effect*, described by Schacter in 1987. Amnesics may also show this priming effect in similar circumstances. In their experiments, Warrington and Weiskrantz (1974) showed that amnesics did as well as normals in the stem completion test, but significantly less well on word recall and recognition tests. This is consistent with the assumption that some memory of the original list was present in amnesics and could be recalled under the right conditions. It would appear that the word-stem completion test provided these subjects with enough cues so that an emotional association was not necessary for retrieval. This seems to support the mechanism proposed for the deficits seen in semantic memory.

But what about the apparent preservation of procedural-type memories in amnesics? In general, this type of memory should also suffer from the absence of a normal emotional drive provided by the hippocampus. In essence, these entities should lack the repetitive reinforcement and contextual emotional reference that normal memories receive from the hippocampus. Like semantic memories, experiential repetition is probably critical for their storage. But unlike semantic memories, very little retrieval failure is usually observed. The explanation for this apparent paradox may actually be relatively simple. Neither form of memory has an emotional association that can aid in retrieval, but procedural memories have a motor component that may substitute for this missing function. For an amnesic to acquire procedural memories, some motor task must be practiced. Through this repetitive process, the memory of the task is stored through continual reinforcement from experience, as described for semantic memories. Unlike semantic memories, the motor movements involved in the learning task would also be stored in the motor cortex and linked in association with the memory of the activity itself.

To perform the learned task, the amnesic is presented with the experimental device. This alone may not be sufficient to trigger the procedural memory. The memory of the device itself would seem to have no more strength than the semantic memory of a word and could be recalled with no more ease. Upon presentation of the device, subjects might manually explore it in such a way as to remind them of the prior learned activity. In other words, certain manual hand movements might serve as a trigger or cue for the memory of the previously rehearsed task. In combination, the motor, visual, and tactile cues might be sufficient to activate the procedural memory and allow the task to be performed, even in the absence of emotional cues. In this example, the cuing information is not emotional, but comes from the random hand manipulation of the experimental device when it is initially presented. This may substitute for the emotional cue and provide enough information for the task to be repeated. The memory of the training sessions themselves might not be recalled because, as episodic memories, they might be less well associated with the motor memories and depend more on an emotional context for retrieval. Enough information might be present to trigger the ability to perform the task but not enough to recall the learning sessions themselves.

The hypothesis presented here seems to provide a reasonable explanation for the memory deficits seen in the amnesia resulting from hippocampal loss. As indicated, the hippocampus may provide an *emotional drive* necessary both for the repetitive activation and the consolidation of a new memory. The emotional component of the memory should also become associated through this process. In the absence of this drive, a memory structure may still receive reinforcement through repetition from experience, but no emotion would become associated. Retrieval, which may depend upon an emotional cue in many cases, would appear very difficult or impossible for such structures. There may simply be too little information from the environment to fully specify and activate the memory in question without the emotional component. When the memory of a motor movement is stored with the primary structure, it may substitute for the emotional cue, allowing retrieval to occur, as may happen with procedural memories. The motor cue may simply add another identifying factor from the environment, allowing the main memory to be more completely specified. This may normally be the role of emotional associations in nonmotor memories.

OTHER THEORIES OF AMNESIA

Through the years, many hypotheses have been proposed attempting to explain the memory loss that occurs in amnesia. Perhaps the most influential theory today suggests that amnesia results when facts and life episodes are not properly registered as new memory, as the result of deficits in storage or consolidation (Squire, Shimamura, & Amaral, 1989; Zola-Morgan & Squire, 1990a). According to this theory, recognition and recall fail simply because such structures are not present for reference within the brain. A second theory, advanced by Schacter (1990), suggests that patients with amnesia store information in a normal manner but are unable to bring such memory into consciousness because of a defect in a general-purpose *consciousness awareness system*. In effect, it is proposed that there is a disconnection between the memories that are lost in amnesia and this hypothetical system, which would normally facilitate their entry into awareness. A third group of hypotheses seems to be intermediate between the first two. This suggests that patients with amnesia are unable to bring contextual information into consciousness and, as a consequence, the recall of associated factual and episodic information also fails (Mayes, 1988; Mayes, Meudell, & Pickering, 1985; Schacter, 1990).

The hypothesis presented here differs significantly form the older ideas that have been proposed. *Of prime importance to this theory is the role of emotion*. It has been argued that this mental entity, which has traditionally been ignored by many in neuroscience, may be essential for the localization of memory, as well as its initial consolidation. This theory also predicts that amnesia may occur in some cases because of failure in the localization of an existing memory, and in others because no viable memory was generated during the initial learning experience.

FACIAL AGNOSIA

The study of memory deficits that result when humans experience brain injury is a complex but potentially rewarding area of research. Unfortunately, such studies are subject to a great many variables, because no two lesions are exactly the same. Lesion size and location, variability in normal brain anatomy, and an inability to reproduce such conditions under standardized laboratory conditions are only a few of the factors that influence the interpretation of data from such studies. Despite this, some lesions produce results that are consistent enough to formulate generalizations about their effects on memory. In this section, bilateral lesions occurring in the occipitotemporal interface, which produce *facial agnosia* (*prosopagnosia*), will be briefly considered.

Patients suffering with prosopagnosia are unable to recognize faces known to them before brain injury. In other words, individuals sustaining such damage are no longer able to visually identify family members or friends, and are often unable to recognize their own images in pictures or mirrors. Such individuals also fail to recognize doctors, nurses, and others whom they repeatedly encounter after the injury (Damasio, Tranel, & Damasto, 1990b). Their inability to store this type of new memory appears similar to patients such as H.M., with medial-temporal-lobe amnesia. In most cases, recognition deficits involve more than just faces. Identification of any object with a specific and unique meaning may fail. For example, such patients are often unable to identify their own car, house, or dog as unique entities. Even so, they still retain the ability to taxonomize such objects without difficulty. For example, they may be able to identify the object within their visual field as a house, but not as *their house*. Even though facial recognition generally fails in individuals with prosopagnosia, specific identification of others is often possible when gait or posture is observed. In addition, identification may also be possible from information entering a different sensory modality. For example, a familiar voice can often trigger recognition of a unique individual when facial appearance, alone, fails.

Despite an inability to consciously recognize faces that were familiar before injury, it has been discovered that patients with facial agnosia often show a large *electrodermal skin conductance* in response to such faces. In contrast, unfamiliar faces produce no reaction (Tranel & Damasio, 1985). This has been interpreted as indicating that the physiological basis for facial recognition is intact at some level below consciousness. It should also be noted that such skin responses do not occur in all patients with prosopagnosia (Bauer, 1986; Newcombe, Young, & DeHaan, 1989). In such patients, this is often attributed to profound perceptual difficulties, although Etcoff, Freeman and Cave (1991) have reported that autonomic recognition can also fail in those without a perceptual defect. There is obviously much to learn about the phenomenon of agnosia.

The ideas proposed in this work suggest that memories are composed of individual associations linked in unique ways to reproduce those events perceived through the senses. Reason suggests that, in most cases, the greater the number of associations linked together to define a memory, the more specificity it should possess. This, of course, is based on the assumption that memories composed of more associations would generally display the highest degree of uniqueness when compared with other entities in storage. As a consequence, if the associated components of a large, well-defined memory complex were removed one by one, a progressive loss in specificity of the complex should occur. As a result, the unique and highly recognizable characteristics of a memory should erode until a generalized form of the memory emerged. This was discussed earlier as the process of GMC formation. Eventually, even these generalized memories should lose their identities as association loss continued. At some point, only small, unconnected memory fragments would remain as the original large memory complex became completely degraded. The individual elements that initially composed the memory would still remain in storage, but the specific *pattern of association*, which defined it as a unique mental entity, would be lost.

AN EXPLANATION FOR FACIAL AGNOSIA

It is proposed here that lesions that produce prosopagnosia effectively separate or isolate the structure of the visual memory from its emotional associations. When the image of a familiar face is perceived, it is matched to the corresponding structure in memory, which was stored through previous contacts with this person. The emotion associated with this memory, however, would not be triggered, because the pathway that connects neurons encoding the physical characteristics of the face with those specifying emotion have been interrupted. Because this important identifying association is missing, recognition of the familiar face would fail. The individual may correctly recognize the image as a face (i.e., the GMC for a face would be triggered), but in the absence of the emotional information, its specific identity would remain hidden.

As indicated earlier, when gait or posture is observed, the specific identify of an individual can often be determined. This is, of course, notable because *such information is also perceived visually*. The obvious question at this point is how some forms of visual information can specify a familiar individual when the image of a face may not be sufficient. There would seem to be at least two possibilities that might explain this seeming paradox. The image of posture or gait may act as an additional association, along with the memory of the face, to more completely specify the memory. In other words, perhaps this information can substitute to some extent for the emotional data, permitting a more complete localization of the memory of the individual. It is also possible that memories of motion or physical orientation may be specific enough by themselves to make recognition possible. Emotional information may not be as necessary when this type of cue is present.

Often specific identification of a known individual is possible from the sound of his or her voice, even when facial appearance is not sufficient. According to the scenario proposed here, the memory of the voice would have its own neural structure with separate linkages to defining emotional associations. When this memory is matched by incoming auditory data, its emotional associations may be activated, allowing the individual to be fully specified. In some cases, patients with prosopagnosia may be able to describe some of the physical characteristics of the individual identified through auditory recognition. The theory presented here suggests that the auditory memory would be linked in association with the visual memory, which could also be accessed via this pathway. In other words, once the auditory memory is specified, electrical energy may be transmitted to the visual memory through this associative link, providing information on the individual's physical description.

EMOTIONAL RESPONSES IN FACIAL AGNOSIA

At least one line of research strongly supports the involvement of emotion in prosopagnosia. In an episode of the public television network series "Nova" ("Stranger in the Mirror," December, 1993), recent studies on patients with this disorder were examined. Of particular note was the observation that male patients who were shown provocative pictures of nude females or beautiful landscapes showed *no emotional reaction*. In contrast, a control group of normal males displayed a level of emotional arousal that was considered normal. *Thus, patients with facial agnosia seem to have somehow lost their ability to experience emotional release when presented visual material that would normally produce such a response.* This is, of course, consistent with the hypothesis presented here that *there is a traumatic division separating the emotional component of a memory from the main structure of its visual image in patients with prosopagnosia.*

OTHER MEMORY DEFICITS

Prosopagnosia is characterized by an inability to recognize faces that were previously familiar and other objects with a personal connotation. As indicated before, such patients may still be able to correctly identify the general category to which the object belongs. For example, they may be unable to specifically identify *their dog,* but they can still define it by its physical image as a dog. In other words, some identifying specificity is obviously lost but certainly not that which allows them to classify the general category to which dogs belong. In a second group of patients with *assorted lesions in the temporal lobe* (Warrington & McCarthy, 1987), even this ability may be lost. When shown a picture of a dog, the ability to define it as *a type of animal* may remain but its specific recognition as a dog may fail. It would appear that, in such patients, an even higher degree of specifying information may be lost as a result of their lesions. The explanation for this phenomenon is consistent with the GMC theory of memory structure proposed here.

THE STRUCTURE OF GENERALIZED
MEMORY COMPLEXES

Within a GMC, there are many levels of complexity. At its most basic level, the GMC for a dog may be composed of neurons that provide the most elemental information about these animals. Perhaps this is simply the association of the word *dog* with its verbal definition as an *animal.* At this level, no visual conceptualization of this animal may exist. At the next level of complexity, these neurons may be collectively linked in association with a crude visual image of a typical dog. In turn, this assemblage of neurons may, as a whole, be linked to even greater defining associations. For example, the type and color of fur seen with various dogs, or common facial and body structures, may be defined by additional associations tied to the basic collection of neurons forming the GMC for a dog. Each addition layer of associations may further define the GMC. At the highest level, specific dogs, known to the individual, may be registered. *Emotion would be associated at this level as a defining parameter.* In prosopagnosia, this portion of the GMC may be stripped away, allowing the individual to still categorize the object as a dog but not as *his or her dog.* Other lesions may damage neural tracts at deeper levels of the GMC, resulting in more loss in specificity. As each layer of GMC is peeled away, the object in question would become less specifically defined. The location of a given lesion would determine at what level this occurred and how much specificity was lost. This may account for the various syndromes of memory loss seen in relatively isolated brain lesions.

FACIAL AGNOSIA AND
MEDIAL-TEMPORAL-LOBE AMNESIA

It is noteworthy that patients with facial agnosia may be unable to identify individuals, such as doctors and nurses, who are repeatedly encountered after the injury (Damasio, 1990). In other words, this appears to be a similar form of memory deficit experienced by patients with bilateral hippocampal damage or resection, as in the patient H.M. *As postulated before, the brain lesions observed in patients with prosopagnosia may be localized to those neural tracts that connect the emotional centers to those structures that encode visual images.* In effect, such damage would disrupt the hippocampal cycle, which may serve to strengthen memories in proportion to the intensity of emotion associated with the visual event to be stored in memory. Because the emotion that would normally be evoked by a stimulating visual image is short-circuited, the emotional drive necessary to consolidate memories via the hippocampus would be blocked. Memories of people encountered on a regular basis would thus be *weak and difficult to retrieve.*

DAMASIO'S IDEAS ON FACIAL AGNOSIA

The explanation for prosopagnosia that is presented here is actually similar to that proposed by Antonio Damasio, who has published extensively on this subject. Damasio conceptualizes memories as consisting of single composite representations that are connected through different channels to each sensory modality (Damasio, Damasio, Tranel, & Brandt, 1990a; Damasio et al., 1990b). In contrast, other authors believe that each sensory modality has its own separate form of representation in memory (McCarthy & Warrington, 1988). Damasio feels that the inability to identify a familiar face is the result of destruction of the visual pathway to the mental representation of this face rather than loss of the memory itself. According to this interpretation, an individual with prosopagnosia may still be able to access this memory through auditory or other sensory channels. This is in complete agreement with the hypothesis presented here.

Damasio also suggests that recognition deficits result when *feedback projections,* which are postulated to link abstract parts of the memory to more concrete forms (*modality-specific representations*), are lesioned (Damasio, 1990). Thus individuals may be able to classify an animal as a dog but may fail to recognize it as *their dog*. He also postulates that lesions in other areas may, in a like manner, produce recognition deficits at other levels. For example, lesions in other areas may prevent identification of an animal as a dog because the feedback projections appropriate for this level of identification have been cut. These ideas are, of course, consistent with the conceptualization presented here, that recognition deficits become more profound as levels of the GMC representing the image are stripped away. In other words, the feedback projections referred to by Damasio may, in fact, be *structural components of GMCs*.

It is also significant that Damasio recognizes *emotion* as a factor that may play a role in recognition (Damasio, 1990). He postulates that if a specific object has a strong positive or negative connotation, its visual image may evoke feelings that may provide affective input to the relevant memory. Such input may thus aid in the recognition of objects with an emotional connotation. Damasio also suggests that a number of other factors, such as *motor patterns characteristic for interaction with a particular object, may serve as recognition cues*. This idea was also proposed earlier in this chapter as a way patients with *medial-temporal-lobe amnesia* may be able to recall motor tasks. *It is suggested here that the destruction of those channels that link a memory with its associated emotion is the main cause for facial agnosia. Such associations may be important memory components that confer categorical specificity.*

THE AMYGDALA

The role of the amygdala in medial-temporal-lobe amnesia remains a controversial subject. In some animal studies, it has been claimed that lesions of the amygdala impair the acquisition of new memory in emotional learning situations (Cahill & McGaugh, 1990; Hitchcock & Davis, 1987; Kesner, Walser, & Winzenried, 1989; LeDoux, Iwata, Cicchetti, & Reis, 1988; Weiskrantz, 1956). In others, experiments have suggested that emotional behavior and new learning are *anatomically dissociable*, and that memory impairment is related to damage of the hippocampus and its anatomically related cortex rather than to conjoint damage of the hippocampus and amygdala (Zola-Morgan, Squire, Alvarez-Royo, & Clower, 1991). From the hypothesis that has been presented here, a role for the amygdala in amnesia and learning can be postulated.

In a previous chapter, the possible existence of *emotional centers* within the brain was considered. These entities may be physically characterized as neural structures that produce the sensation of emotion for the brain when activated. Research has demonstrated that a wide range of emotion can be elicited by the electrical stimulation of various brain regions, which presumably contain emotional centers or neural projections that lead to such structures. It has been postulated here that such centers are electrically connected to structures that encode memory and serve as associations that impart meaning. The amygdala is a brain structure associated with aversive learning and conditioned fear. It is known that electrical stimulation of the amygdala *alone* will produce the perception of fear in animals, as judged by changes in behavior, as well as in humans (Davis, 1992). In addition, animals with selective damage to this structure display a reduced level of fear in novel situations (Zola-Morgan et al., 1991). *It is therefore postulated here that the amygdala represents an emotional center that is specific for the sensation of fear.* It may be anatomically prominent because fear is a common emotion upon which survival depends. It is conceivable that other emotional centers may be smaller and less anatomically obvious because of the relative importance of the emotion they convey.

In the work by Zola-Morgan and associates (1991), the relationship of temporal lobe damage to emotional behavior was examined in monkeys. These animals show patterns of amnesia that are similar in many ways to those displayed by humans (Zola-Morgan & Squire, 1990b). Emotional scores were based on the animals' reactions to seven inanimate objects that were selected to elicit investigatory or consummatory behavior. Ten minutes later, memory for the learning situation was tested. Groups tested included control animals without brain damage, animals with damage to the both the hippocampal formation and the amygdala, animals with lesions of the hippocampal formation but not the amygdala, and animals with damage to the hippocampal formation and associated cortical areas but not the amygdala. It was found that amygdala damage affected only emotional behavior, without detectable changes in memory. In contrast, animals with only hippocampal injury showed impairment in memory but not in emotional response. Animals with lesions of both areas showed deficits in both memory and emotional reaction. From these data it was concluded that emotional behavior and memory impairment are anatomically dissociable. *On the surface*, these data seem to suggest that memory storage is independent of emotion.

The hypothesis presented here suggests that selectively removing or lesioning the amygdala may affect *only new memory, which becomes associated with fear.* Even so, such selective damage may not eliminate learning completely. It is likely that emotion, *other than fear*, arising from undamaged emotional centers, may also be stimulated by the learning situation, allowing some emotional association and memory acquisition to occur. It has been a recurring theme throughout this work that emotions rarely exist alone as single entities within the brain. In almost all situations, a blend of emotions is probably necessary to fully define and interpret ongoing events. Experiments in which the amygdala is lesioned may therefore *not truly reflect a dissociation of emotion from learning.* Such conditions may only eliminate a single emotion, without affecting others that might also be stimulated, and be capable of driving new memory storage. Under such conditions, learning might appear normal, especially if the conditions of the experiment did not evoke appreciable amounts of fear, as appears to be the case in the work presented by Zola-Morgan and associates (1991).

It is probably significant that the cortical areas surrounding the hippocampus (the perirhinal and parahippocampal cortices), which were lesioned in the Zola-Morgan et al. experiments, were also found to be important for the acquisition of new memory (also see Clower, Zola-Morgan, & Squire, 1990; Squire & Zola-Morgan, 1991; Zola-Morgan, Squire, Amaral, & Suzuki, 1989). These areas are known to provide the majority of input to the hippocampus from the neocortex (Insausti, Amaral, & Cowan, 1987) and, as such, may contain other emotional centers or projections from such structures leading to the hippocampus. Damage to these areas may interrupt input from *many* emotional centers and therefore produce a more profound memory impairment than destruction of the amygdala alone. Under such experimental conditions, virtually all emotional input may be attenuated, resulting in gross memory impairment.

The role of the amygdala in emotional learning has been strengthened by the work of LeDoux (1986, 1990). Employing fear-conditioning experiments in rats, this researcher has demonstrated a subcortical pathway that mediates this process when an auditory signal is used as the conditioned stimulus. It was found that acoustical inputs are transmitted through the auditory system to the level of the medial geniculate body (MGB). At this point, the posterior intralaminar nucleus (a structure adjacent to and possibly related to the medial division of the MGB) relays the signal on to the lateral nucleus of the amygdala and then to the amygdala's central nucleus (ACE). It was found that projections from the ACE to the hypothalamus were involved in autonomic conditioned responses (as changes in blood pressure or heart rate), and those that led to central gray areas of the brain controlled the expression of conditioned emotional behavior such as freezing. The finding that this pathway operates below the level of the neocortex strengthens Izard's contention (see Chapter 5 for a discussion of this) that some emotion can arise in the absence of true cognition. It is further suggested by LeDoux that through reciprocal connections with the hippocampus, the amygdala may also be involved in fear conditioning, which is more cognitive in nature. It is also of note that the visual pathways that mediate aversive learning have been studied by Davis (1992).

CONCLUDING REMARKS

In this chapter, *amnesia is considered to be a state-dependent effect*. Memory recall may fail because emotions in the prevailing mood do not adequately support the localization of those memories associated with other emotions. Such effects may explain the memory losses that accompany the various dissociative disorders, and those that arise from hippocampal removal. Central to this proposal is the concept that emotions may serve as important retrieval cues. In the absence of appropriate emotion, memory localization may fail, and amnesia may result. The ideas presented here appear quite different from those of earlier theories, which have attempted to explain dissociation phenomena (Schacter, 1989) and amnesia (McClelland & Rumelhart, 1986; Wickelgren, 1979).

Association Hypothesis and Mood Disorders

A theory is presented in this chapter that attempts to link depression and mania with the association hypothesis. It is suggested that both mental disorders arise from a common mechanism involving a disruption in the normal balance between memories and their associated emotions. This hypothesis represents a logical extension of ideas and concepts presented in earlier chapters.

BACKGROUND

Over the years, many hypotheses have been proposed to explain depression. Perhaps the earliest of these was based upon the psychoanalytic theory (Newman & Hirt, 1983) originated by Freud. This proposal was based on the idea that repressed memories and emotions could emerge at later times to produce the symptoms of depression. Others theories have suggested that depression is a cognitive response to the negative features in life (Beck et al., 1979). In effect, some aspects of this illness may actually be learned. A variation of this model suggests that depression is a state of learned helplessness occurring in response to overwhelming life circumstances (Peterson & Seligman, 1984). Biological theories of depression as well as mania have often focused on chemical changes which may occur in the synaptic junctions which link neurons (Janowsky, El-Yousef, & Davis, 1972; Murphy, Campbell, & Costa, 1978; Schildkraut, 1965). It has been proposed that mood changes and depression may result when one or more of the neurotransmitters that mediate cellular communication are lost. In support of this idea is the observation that most antidepressant medications block the reuptake of neurotransmitters at synaptic junctions, producing a relative increase in the concentration of these substances. Much speculation has also centered on the neuroendocrine changes and sleep disturbances that often accompany affective disorders (Georgotas & Cancro, 1988; Reynolds & Kupfer, 1988). Each of these theories views depression from a different perspective and all seem to provide some insight into this mental affliction. The extreme complexity of mood disorders suggests that there may be many valid ways of approaching this difficult subject. The hypothesis proposed in this chapter is based upon the associative nature of memory and emotion. Since Kraepelin originally noted that rhymes and sound associations increase during mania, several investigators have suggested that associative patterns may change during episodes of depression and mania (Henry, Weingartner, & Murphy, 1971; Kraepelin, 1921/ 1976; Murphy, 1923).

In this hypothesis, it is assumed that the emotion associated with memory is not static but may gradually change upon exposure to different moods. This may occur because a memory passing through consciousness may release its associated emotion into the mood to provide interpretation for the activated memory and also associate with those emotions present in the current mood, which were acquired from other memories during prior interpretative rounds. A memory passing through consciousness may therefore donate as well as acquire new emotion. The mood might thus be viewed as a repository for emotion, allowing it to be transferred from one memory to the next. This important concept is illustrated in Figure 8.1.

If a memory that acquired emotion from a given mood is recalled at some later time, the emotion released during its interpretation may enter consciousness and, in part, reproduce the original mood that provided the associated emotion. In this way, an existing emotional tone may be carried forward to color the composition of future moods. This reciprocal exchange of associated emotion between recalled memories and existing moods may constitute a mechanism that is basic to consciousness. Support for this concept will be presented in various ways and from different perspectives throughout this chapter. It is suggested that this basic process is central to the generation and maintenance of mood disorders.

The mechanism described, by which emotion is transferred to thoughts cycling through consciousness, is conceptually consistent with other aspects of the association hypothesis that have been presented.

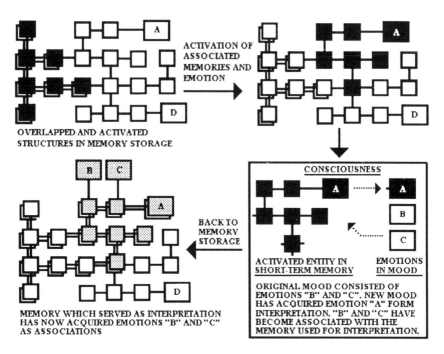

Figure 8.1 In the upper-left portion of this figure, a structure in memory storage is overlapped by incoming data, and an associated memory containing emotion A is activated. This memory and its associated emotion enter consciousness to serve as an interpretation for the original data. Emotion A becomes part of the mood, and the memory liberated during this process associates with emotion already present in the mood from previous rounds of interpretation. The mood thus serves as a repository for emotion that is released during interpretation and as a source of new emotion for memories passing through consciousness.

Emotion in the mood and memories in consciousness each seem to represent mental perceptions arising from the activation of underlying neural structures. According to Hebb's ideas, if such neural complexes are activated simultaneously, or in close temporal succession, they should be subject to some degree of association. These concepts suggest that the transfer of emotion from the mood to memories cycling through consciousness may actually be an associative phenomenon that may normally occur as underlying structures are activated during the initial matching and localization process. The resulting strength of association is probably directly related to the temporal proximity of such activations. In other words, those structures that undergo rapid activation to produce perceptions that enter consciousness in close succession may normally experience a greater degree of association with each other than those that are temporally more separated. An exception to this may occur when an emotion is intense and remains in consciousness for extended periods of time. Under such conditions, memories entering consciousness at much later times may still be exposed to a sufficient intensity of emotion to produce some association. In other words, the temporal proximity of activated structures, as well as the intensity of emotion remaining in the mood from prior interpretations, may each influence the strength of association that ultimately results. In subsequent paragraphs, these concepts will be considered in relationship to the generation of mood disorders.

POLARIZED EMOTION

When stimulating life events occur, prolonged moods consisting of intense emotion may result. Under these conditions, more memories than normal may associate with emotion from the resulting mood because of its enduring presence. The normal balance between memories and associated emotions may eventually become shifted through this process. In other words, the distribution of emotional associations may become skewed or polarized, reflecting the mood generated by the stimulating events. During the subsequent use of such memories in thought, the original mood should again be reproduced to some extent through the release of this emotion during the interpretative process. If the degree of polarization was extensive (i.e., if a substantial number of memories in current usage acquired a single type of emotional presence), recall of such memories in routine thought might serve to continuously regenerate the original mood state. Such conditions may favor the establishment of affective disorders by producing prolonged moods from which escape is difficult.

When a preponderance of memories used in current thought acquires associated emotion from an intense and prolonged mood, shifts to other mood states containing different emotions should become difficult and less frequent. Under these conditions, many memories passing through consciousness should perpetuate the original mood state to some extent. In addition, such memories should also experience an increase in synaptic strength through the polarization process, which should enhance their retention in consciousness and further prolong the mood. This important concept will be discussed later in this chapter. Over time, a single mood might thus become fixed and dominant through these mental changes. At this point, generation of the original mood would no longer be restricted exclusively to recollections of those events that produced the original parent mood. Many peripherally related memories that received polarized emotion should also be capable of reproducing this mood to some extent. It is conceivable that the narrowed range of moods that seem characteristic of depression and mania may originate in this manner. This will be discussed in subsequent paragraphs.

It is proposed that both depression and mania may result when an increased proportion of memories used in current thought acquire emotional components of the same or closely related type. Such associative changes may produce a dominant state of emotional polarization, which

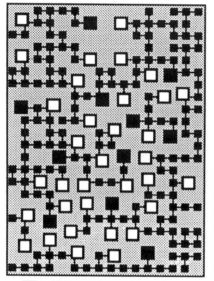
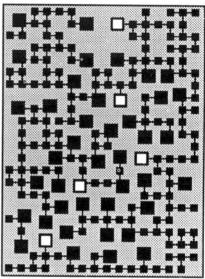

FIELD OF MEMORIES DISPLAYING HETEROGENOUS ASSOCIATED EMOTION WHICH WOULD PRODUCE A NORMAL (EUTHYMIC) MOOD AS THE RESULT OF MEMORY INTERPRETATION.

FIELD OF MEMORIES DISPLAYING POLARIZED EMOTION WHICH WOULD PRODUCE A MOOD COMPATIBLE WITH DEPRESSION OR MANIA.

Figure 8.2 Small, black squares represent neurons, whereas large, black-and-white squares symbolize associated emotions, which are opposite in type. For example, black squares may represent anger, hate, sadness, fear, or any number of negative emotions, whereas white squares may symbolize joy, love, pleasure, and similar positive emotions. The memory field on the left represents a normal blend of associated emotion, which would produce euthymic moods as the result of memory interpretation. In contrast, the right memory field is polarized, in that it contains a predominance of negative emotion. Such a grouping of memories would produce a dysphoric mood through memory interpretation, which would be characteristic of depression or dysphoric mania.

may generate and perpetuate the pathological moods that exist in these illnesses. Under normal conditions, it is suggested that thoughts and memories that are cycled through consciousness during routine thinking acquire a variety of emotions from different moods. As these memories are subsequently recalled during routine mental activity, a balanced array of moods would normally be generated. This may not be the case in depression and mania. In these disorders, a redistribution of emotional associations may occur in response to one or more emotionally stimulating life events. A disruption in the normal balance of mood states may eventually result when interpretations are based on memories associated with polarized emotion. Figure 8.2 represents a conceptualization of polarized and normal memory fields.

From general observation, the number of moods experienced in depression and mania seems relatively small. In other words, the wide range of moods seen in nonpathological conditions seems to be dramatically reduced in these illnesses. This appears to be generally characteristic of mood disorders. As each illness progresses, the range of potential moods seems to narrow. Eventually a representative emotional presence emerges, which characterizes the disorder in question. For example, the typical depressed state may consist of various proportions of despair, sorrow, fear, anxiety, anger, frustration, and other similar feelings, which cumulatively produce a dominate emotional tone. In full-blown depression, a mood representative of some combination of these emotions is essentially present all of the time. Positive emotion is experienced less often as the illness intensifies. The wide diversity of normally available moods seems to diminish. A limited number of mood states also seems to characterize mania.

DEPRESSION AND MANIA AS SUBSETS
OF THE SAME ILLNESS

It is proposed that both depression and mania arise from the same basic mechanism. The primary difference between the two states may be the type of emotion that becomes polarized. In a sense, both conditions might be considered to be subsets of the same general illness. If negative emotions become spread to other memories, depression may result. If emotions with a more positive or energized flavor become involved, mania may appear. The state that ultimately develops is probably dependent upon the particular life circumstances experienced at any given time and the individual's perception of these conditions. Both states seem to represent a severe imbalance in the normal distribution of associated emotions.

The suggestion that depression and mania are each manifestations of the same basic illness is supported by clinical research utilizing lithium. This metallic ion, in its carbonate or citrate salt form, has proven to be highly effective in the treatment of mania and the mood lability characteristic of affective disorders. The usefulness of this medication for psychiatric illness was originally suggested in the 1940s by the work of John Cade, an Australian state hospital superintendent. Since then, this mood stabilizer has become widely used for the treatment of a number of psychiatric conditions. In two large-scale studies performed in the 1960s and 1970s (Angst, Weis, Baastrup, & Schou, 1970; Baastrup & Schou, 1967), lithium was found to be as effective for the prevention of depression as it is for mania. This, of course, suggests that these two psychiatric conditions may have a common biological basis, as suggested in the hypothesis presented here.

To better understand these ideas, perhaps it would be helpful to consider in more detail the mechanism by which a mood disorder may develop. Although depression will be illustrated here, the same general principles probably also apply to mania. As indicated before, both disorders may evolve from the same underlying mechanism, but the nature of the precipitating events and the emotions that become fixated may vary widely.

THE EVOLUTION OF DEPRESSION

In many cases, an episode of major depression may be preceded by an unexpected, tragic life event. This might provide the seed for the process to begin by establishing a dominant, negative emotional tone. Memories and emotions surrounding the event might remain in consciousness for relatively long periods of time. Initially, a core of memories closely related to the situation would acquire negative emotion from the mood. The process of polarization would have begun. If the mood were intense and prolonged, the spread of negative emotion to other memories might continue and become extensive. Over time, most people in such a situation may be capable of experiencing enough positive emotion to prevent the negative background from becoming totally dominant. Events that stimulate positive or other types of emotion should allow a wider variety of moods to be experienced and offset the exclusive spread of negative emotion. Enough balance may be maintained in the prevailing mood state to prevent the development of a major depression. In a small percentage of people, the situation might be overwhelming, or their ability to cope with adversity might be inadequate. They might be incapable of generating enough opposing emotion to effectively counter the transfer of negative feelings. Over time, many memories might become associated with dysphoric emotion, and the normal emotional balance would be destroyed. Negative moods would predominate and major depression would develop.

These ideas suggest that depression may involve changes in the normal association patterns of memories and emotions. Under normal circumstances, a dynamic equilibrium involving a variety of different mood states probably exists. The entities that compose this system are probably in a constant state of flux, reflecting current experience. Small disruptions in this balance are probably normal and may occur frequently as different events alter the current emotional emphasis. Under these conditions, the number of mood states generally available is probably large because of the wide variety of emotions associated with memories used in current thought. No single mood would be excessively dominant or prolonged. Excessive and lasting shifts in this normal dynamic emotional balance may result in pathological mood states.

In depression, there may be a large shift in the normal distribution of memories and their associated emotions. The process may begin when a few memories central to a current situation acquire a dominant negative emotion. This may occur slowly, as described, or more rapidly, if the involved events are acute and intense. Over time, negative emotion may spread from the mood to many other less directly related memories. A high degree of emotional polarization, involving many current memories, may eventually result. In effect, many memories of current interest may acquire a complement of negative emotion. Under such conditions, a prolonged dysphoric mood should be generated by the emotional interpretations that arise from the use of these memories in routine thought. In this way, the dysphoric mood of depression would be propagated.

Once begun, the process leading to depression would be self-perpetuating. As more memories acquired negative emotion, the dominant emotional tone would become increasingly negative, and the process would become accelerated. The patient would progressively lose the capacity to experience positive emotion as negative associations became dominant. It might occur slowly at first, when the emotional tone was only slightly negative. Without the input of significant positive emotion to restore the balance by changing the mood, the negative decline would continue. In most cases, some pleasurable emotion would be present to slow the process. Eventually many memories of current interest would become associated to some extent with dysphoric emotion. A state of emotional polarization involving an increased proportion of memories in current usage would result. Dysphoria, unpleasant feelings, and anxiety would be continually generated from ongoing mental interpretation. The overall emotional tone would be negative. The transfer of this type of emotion, through the mechanism proposed, may be a factor in the development of some forms of depression.

The described negative decline in emotional status might continue for weeks to months for a significant depression to develop. True depression appears to be a global change in mental status, which does not occur instantly. At any point during the emotional decline, a change in life circumstances might produce enough positive emotion to arrest or reverse the process by generating opposing moods. After several months, untreated depression will usually remit. Once improvement starts, the same extended time course may be observed. Several months may be required for complete recovery, regardless of the type of treatment employed. Obviously, some process is occurring, which requires the passage of time. It is conceivable that healing requires a reassociation of positive or at least nonnegative emotion with the many memories contributing to depression. In effect, recovery may require another redistribution of emotional associations.

SYMPTOMS OF DEPRESSION AND MANIA

The type of emotion that becomes fixed in depression may explain many of the symptoms common to this disorder. For example, the slowness of thought and the perception of extreme fatigue may in part arise from the deenergizing nature of the emotions that characterize this condition. There may simply be no emotional drive to support normal thought and activity. The helpless and hopeless feelings frequently reported may be natural cognitive responses to such an intractable mental state. To some extent, the memory and concentration problems seen in depression may also be a consequence of this slowed cognitive state. In contrast, energizing emotions seem to dominate in mania. These may run the gamut from anger to pure euphoria. Almost any combination of feelings may be seen in this disorder. The presence of emotion in polarized form may provide the incredible drive in thought and behavior, which seems to characterize mania.

Although mania is often described as an expansive and euphoric state, which is the opposite of depression, in reality, moods composed of many different emotions may actually be present in the active phase of this illness. In 1969, Winokur, Clayton, and Reich observed depressive symptoms in 68% of a study group composed of 100 manic patients. Roughly similar results were found in a 1971 study by Beigel and Murphy (1974) in which they concluded (p. 647) that the equation of elated mood with mania represents an oversimplification of the varied phenomena of mania. They further suggested that mania might best be described as a state of heightened overall activation, rather than elation. Although depression is generally considered to be a state of pervasive negative emotion, it would appear that some forms of mania may be almost indistinguishable from depression and differ only in the degree of emotional drive that is displayed. It is proposed here that the type and nature of emotion that become dominant and fixed in the mood of manic–depressive patients determine the phase of illness observed.

Patients suffering from severe depression often seem unable to recall pleasurable memories. Such entities simply do not seem available for reference. Memory retrieval problems may be widespread and are a frequent complaint in depressed patients. With only a limited number of mood states available, state-dependent effects may become noticeable. This concept was introduced in a previous chapter. The localization and retrieval of memories not associated with the depressed mood state may be difficult or impossible. In depression, partial or complete amnesia for such memories may be experienced. The focus of all mental activity would be consistent with the dominant dysphoric state, effectively excluding the recall of memories associated with other moods. These ideas are supported by studies indicating that depressed patients are better able to recall words that evoke negative emotion, whereas nondepressed subjects show the opposite effect (Davis, 1979a, 1979b; Kuiper & Derry, 1982). Depressed patients are also more likely to recall unpleasant experiences than those with a more positive emotional content (Fogarty & Hemsley, 1983; Lloyd & Lishman, 1975).

In mania, memory deficits seem less evident but may also be present. Manic individuals often have such a strong emotional drive that memories inconsistent with the current mood state seem to be of little concern. It seems probable that memory deficits are also present but less noticeable in the energized state, which characterizes true mania. The extreme lack of insight that often characterizes this mental state may represent a deficiency in memory. As in depression, some inability to properly access memories associated with other moods would be predicted by the hypothesis presented here. The state-dependent nature of mania is supported by studies done in 1977 by Weingartner, Miller, and Murphy. These researchers found that patients who cycled between manic and normal states were able to recall verbal associations most efficiently in the same state in which learning originally occurred. In other words, associations established during manic episodes were more easily recalled during mania than in more normal conditions of mood. Information learned during normal mood states also showed the same selectivity. These authors concluded that the mood state influences both memory storage and recall.

In early depression, some ability to shift into alternate mood states for brief periods of time may remain. This would be expected before the narrowed range of moods became completely dominant. As a consequence, recall of memories associated with other moods might still be possible to some extent. There might be only a marginal impairment of memory and concentration noted at this point. As the illness progressed, achieving and maintaining alternate moods might become more difficult. A more profound effect on concentration and the ability to sustain a rational chain of thought would be observed. The patient might have difficulty completing sentences or properly responding to questions if the mood states necessary for such functions could not be maintained for a reasonable time. Memory localization and retrieval would obviously be impaired under such conditions. Thought blocking and confused speech might become apparent. A general state of mental disorganization would exist. These symptoms are frequently observed in severe depression. The inability to maintain appropriate mood states for adequate periods of time may thus impair all functions requiring concentration. This would, of course, also include the ability to store new memory.

As indicated before, the slowness of thought, speech, and physical movement (collectively known as psychomotor retardation), which often seems to characterize depression (Carlson & Strober, 1979; Winokur et al., 1969), may reflect the deenergizing nature of emotions that dominate consciousness. They simply may not provide the emotional drive necessary for normal activity. In contrast, the nature of emotions that characterize mania may be quiet different. As a consequence, thoughts and speech may race, and physical activity may be energetic. Obviously, neural cells, mediating such contrasting levels of mental activity, should differ in their basic requirements for energy. Perhaps this explains the remarkable positron emission tomographic (PET) brain scans published by Baxter et al. in 1985. In this study, a rapid-cycling, manic–depressive patient was found to utilize significantly less metabolic glucose during periods of depression than hypomania.

A loss of interest in normal activities is a frequent complaint associated with depression. Patients may no longer derive pleasure from the numerous simple events that give life its fullness and meaning. In part, such mental changes may result from the association of negative emotion with activities that were formerly enjoyable. Such a global loss of interest might also arise from an inability to concentrate and sustain coherent thought. It may simply be too difficult to maintain the level of interest necessary to engage in normal activities. Routine daily tasks may become viewed as insurmountable. Thought itself may become burdensome. The enormous energy required to maintain an alternate mood state through concentration may produce overwhelming fatigue. Depressed patients often report that they feel mentally drained and do not have the energy for the simplest activities. These may be cognitive responses to the enormous effort required to maintain even marginal levels of normal thought and mental function.

Severe depression has been characterized as a state of mood inflexibility. As recovery occurs, presumably the skewed pattern of emotional associations responsible for this condition becomes normalized. As this occurs, a more normal degree of mood flexibility should also return. As a consequence, concentration and memory retrieval should again become possible as different mood states become available. In ideal situations, the process should continue until normal mental function and mood are completely restored. In effect, a normal distribution of emotional associations reflecting life circumstances would be reestablished.

CATATONIC DEPRESSION

In a small fraction of patients, severe depression may culminate in catatonia. Such individuals are usually mute and totally incapable of caring for themselves. There is generally little, if any, evidence of productive mental activity. The mechanism presented here suggests that a mood state compatible with depression may become totally fixed and inescapable at this point. Under these conditions, the brain may be totally amnestic for all memories except those associated with the single, dominant mood. No other emotional states would be available. The range of possible mental activities would therefore be severely restricted. Speech would fail, because there would literally be nothing to say. The ideas and thoughts normally expressed in words would largely be absent from consciousness. Their retrieval would not be possible, because the mood states required for localization could not be generated. All other normal activities would be suspended for the same reason. Mental activity would truly be fragmented. Normal mental function may require the participation of hundreds or perhaps thousands of individual mood states. In catatonia, this number may be close to unity. Under such conditions, a dramatic loss in function would be expected.

It has long been known that temporary relief from catatonia can be achieved by the intravenous administration of sodium amobarbital (Dysken, 1979). This is commonly referred to as an amytal interview. Under the influence of this barbiturate, the ability to verbally communicate and express ideas is partially restored. Catatonia returns when the procedure is terminated. This observation supports the state-dependent view of this phenomenon. As previously suggested, a wide variety of drugs may have the ability to change or influence the dominant emotional state. Sodium amobarbital may alter the fixed mood existing in catatonia, allowing other emotional states to be expressed. Localization of memories associated with these states would thus become possible, allowing a temporary resumption of some mental function.

It is proposed that the catatonia occurring in depression is a direct consequence of the mood intractability that seems to characterize this disorder. The administration of sodium amobarbital may allow the expression of other emotions and moods, thus permitting the localization and expression of memories not associated with the dominant depressed condition. In a previous chapter, it was suggested that functional or psychogenic amnesia may also arise when mood states become fixed. If these two conditions do, in fact, share this common mechanism, then sodium amobarbital should also support memory recall in functional amnesia. This is exactly what is seen clinically. Sodium amobarbital and similar drugs will often stimulate the recall of lost memories in this form of amnesia (Kaplan & Sadock, 1988; Ruedrich, Chu, & Wadle, 1985). It may also be significant that this barbiturate has proven to be clinically useful for retrieving inaccessible memories in multiple personality disorder (Hall, LeCann, & Schoolar, 1978; Marcos & Trujillo, 1978; Naples & Hackett, 1978). These observations support the concept that depression and amnesia may both involve an inflexibility in mood states.

It has been proposed that depression and mania are mental states that differ primarily in the type of emotion that becomes fixed in consciousness. It has also been suggested that catatonic depression is a consequence of the mood inflexibility that may characterize this condition. Based upon this reasoning, catatonia should also occur in mania. This has been observed clinically (Abrams & Taylor, 1981; Taylor & Abrams, 1977). The occurrence of catatonia in mania provides support for the contention that both depression and mania may each originate and be maintained through a common mechanism. Perhaps at some point in the course of each condition, a prevailing mood becomes so intractable that escape is virtually impossible, and a state of catatonia results.

THE HIPPOCAMPUS AND MOOD DISORDERS

A general theoretical construct has been proposed that attempts to link depression and mania with the association hypothesis. It is suggested that both mental disorders arise from the redistribution of emotional associations with memories. Such skewed associative changes may perpetuate the abnormal mood states seen in these conditions. By examining ideas developed earlier in this work, this general concept can be expanded and viewed in relationship to normal mental function. In the following paragraphs, a possible relationship between the hippocampus and the generation of mood disorders will be proposed.

When stimulating events occur, emotion is generated as a form of interpretation. This is part of the normal evaluation process to which all new information is subjected. The intensity and duration of the resulting emotion often seem to parallel the significance associated with the situation. Events of high relevance generally produce emotions that are intense and may last for extended times. In contrast, many events may be perceived as routine and produce only transient rises in emotional intensity. This rise and fall in emotion repeats itself so frequently and spontaneously that it usually attracts little attention. It is accepted as a common and normal part of mental life. This general phenomenon may be related to hippocampal function and the generation of mood disorders, as will be discussed.

In the preceding chapter, it was suggested that the hippocampus responds to emotion to produce memory consolidation. The degree of reinforcement received by a new memory may be proportional to the intensity of the emotion driving the process. The ultimate strength of a memory would therefore parallel its perceived emotional significance. In this way, events of importance would produce stronger and more lasting memories. This would have obvious biological significance for the brain.

It is suggested that the normal rise and fall in emotion that occur in response to stimulating events may involve the hippocampal mechanism described. In effect, the hippocampus may influence the duration of emotional responses that arise during the interpretative process. When events occur that produce an elevation in emotional intensity, hippocampal activity may be stimulated. Once begun, the process would be propagated by emotion released during the repetitive firing of the involved memories. Reinforcement of the new structures would continue as long as emotional intensity remained high. As a consequence, such memories and their emotional associations would remain in the forefront of the brain as long as the process continued. With intensely emotional situations, the manifestations of the underlying process might be obvious. Hippocampal activity would be high and, as a consequence, memories and feelings associated with the stimulating events would seem to remain in, or close to, consciousness for relatively long periods of time. Thinking would be dominated by thoughts and recollections of the situation. There would literally be a preoccupation with memories and emotions surrounding the stimulating situation. In contrast, events of a more routine nature would produce only a transient rise in hippocampal activity and quickly pass from active awareness. The role of the hippocampus would be less obvious in such cases. The focus of mental activity would be less fixed, and the flow of thought would be more flexible.

Such a process would serve at least two important functions. This arrangement should allow events designated as emotionally important to be maintained in the forefront of the brain until they could be dealt with adequately. If events important to survival or the maintenance of normal function were quickly forgotten, the consequences might obviously be serious. A second benefit to this process was alluded to earlier. Events perceived as important would produce strong and lasting memories from the intense emotional drive. Future reference to such memories would therefore be facilitated if similar events were again encountered.

It has been suggested that new memories undergo consolidation via repetitive activation. This may occur when events repeat themselves in experience, or as the result of hippocampal activity. In the absence of the hippocampus, intense emotion could still be experienced, but when the stimulating events ended, the situation would soon fade from consciousness. This general pattern appears to occur in individuals who have sustained bilateral loss or extensive damage in these paired structures. It is proposed that continued hippocampal activity may serve to maintain emotion and memories in or close to active consciousness for perhaps long periods of time after such stimulating events end. Without this mental function, the memories and emotions associated with the death of a loved one or the birth of a child would endure in consciousness no longer than the average trivial occurrence. Such an arrangement would blur the distinction between major and minor events. Important memories would be stored with no more strength than those of less emotional significance. On future recall of such memories, it might be difficult to distinguish events with the most prior relevance.

EMOTIONAL DILUTION

As suggested here, hippocampal activity may continue until the emotion associated with a stimulating event decreases in intensity. It is postulated that this may occur through a process that is referred to here as emotional dilution. As indicated, repetitive activation of a new memory by the hippocampus during the consolidation process should produce frequent release of the involved emotion into the mood. Here it should mix with other emotions present, producing a blended emotional tone, as discussed earlier. Memories of the precipitating events passing through consciousness would combine with this blended emotion and, once again, return to memory storage. Each cycle through consciousness would alter the associated emotional complement to some extent. In effect, the original associated emotion would become progressively diluted with emotion from the mood on each passage through consciousness. At some point, sufficient emotional dilution would be achieved to slow or terminate the hippocampal drive. Subjectively, the emotions of the original events would become progressively blunted by this process, and recall of the precipitating events would become less frequent. Slowly the events, which were so dominant a short time before, would pass from active awareness. The mental fixation produced by repetitive hippocampal activation would wane as emotion became sufficiently diluted. Other issues of concern would return to consciousness, and the focus of mental activity would shift.

The process described would provide the brain with a way of dissipating strong emotion. As long as hippocampal activity continued, intense emotion would be brought into consciousness, and would mix with other emotions present in the mood. Such emotion would then be picked up by other thoughts and memories passing through consciousness. In effect, an exchange of emotion between memories should occur, as suggested earlier. The strong emotion, originally associated with a few specific memories, would become diluted by the acquisition of new emotion from other memories that passed through consciousness. In this way, concentrated emotion may be dissipated by the process of emotional dilution. The role of the hippocampus in the process of emotional dilution is illustrated in Figure 8.3.

When the high frequency of emotionally stimulating events in life is considered, it seems likely that a large number of separate hippocampal cycles may operate simultaneously at any given time. Some may be transient and short-lived, whereas others may arise from intensely stimulating events and continue for days or longer. Each cycle may contribute some emotion to the prevailing mood, which would be perceived as a single, dominant emotional tone. Changes in emotional focus occurring over time would produce corresponding alterations in mood composition. This may be the normal way moods are created and maintained. Since a wide variety of emotion would be involved in most cases, the overall trend would be toward emotional dilution. In effect, emotion in the current mood would be distributed to a wide range of memories. If, however, a number of emotionally similar events were present in cur-

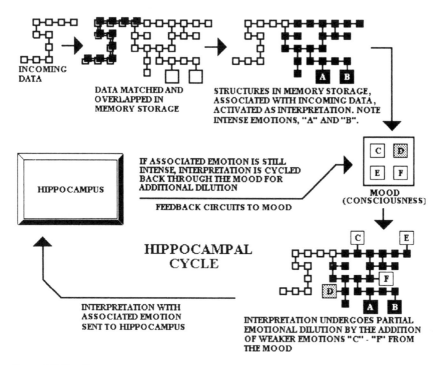

Figure 8.3 Small squares represent neurons, and larger squares symbolize emotions. In the upper-left corner of this figure, incoming data undergo localization in memory storage. As a result, a memory, associated with intense emotions A and B, is activated and enters consciousness as an interpretation for the original data. In the mood, this interpretation associates with emotions (C–F), derived from previous interpretations. The addition of these emotions produces some emotional dilution, thus decreasing somewhat the intensity of emotions A and B associated with the new interpretation. This partially diluted interpretation then travels to the hippocampus, where the level of emotion is sensed and, if it is still intense, the cycle is repeated. This process may go on for many repetitions over time (perhaps weeks to years), until the associated emotion of the interpretation is significantly diluted. In some pathological conditions (such as posttraumatic stress disorder), dilution may never successfully occur, and the individual may suffer emotional pain for many years. It should also be pointed out that the mood is characterized here as containing a variety of relatively weak, different emotions. In states such as depression and mania, the mood may be polarized with like emotion, and interpretations that pass through consciousness (the mood) may become polarized rather than diluted, thus intensifying the pathological state. The status of the mood is, of course, a reflection of the interpretations that pass through it. Emotion held in memory storage can influence the mood through its release into consciousness during interpretation and, in turn, the mood can affect the type and intensity of emotion that returns to and is registered in memory storage.

rent experience, polarization, rather than dilution, might occur. Many memories passing through consciousness might acquire emotion of a similar type. Rather than dilution, the distribution of emotion might become skewed, and a relatively fixed mood state might eventually result. The concepts of emotional dilution and polarization are illustrated in Figure 8.4.

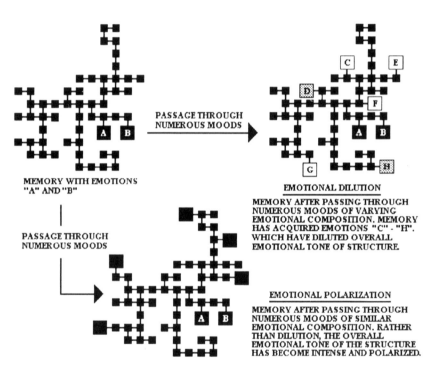

Figure 8.4 In this figure, the concepts of emotional dilution and polarization are illustrated. Small, black squares represent neurons, and larger squares symbolize emotional associations. The figure at the top-left shows a memory associated with emotions A and B. Such emotions would be sensed in consciousness upon memory activation. After multiple passages through different moods of varying emotional composition, new emotions, C–H, are acquired. In this example, these emotions are characterized as relatively weak and opposite A and B. Upon activation, this memory would now produce a relatively neutral blend of emotion. In effect, the original emotion has undergone dilution as a result of this process. In the bottom figure, the original memory has passed through numerous moods with similar emotional content, such as that postulated to exist in depression or mania. It has acquired emotional associations similar to A and B and upon activation, produces intense and polarized emotion. Note that dilution and polarization are produced by the same mechanism and depend upon the emotional composition of the mood through which memories pass.

The hippocampal mechanism proposed may help to understand how the distribution of emotional associations may become skewed in mood disorders. If a number of dysphoric events occurred in current experience, a predominance of negative emotion might flood the mood and be passed on to other memories. Rather than emotional dilution, a concentration of negative emotion would result. If this continued for an extended time, the polarization of such associations might become so extensive as to produce a self-perpetuating, negative mood state. A full-blown depression would be the result. It is also conceivable that a single, very intense, negative experience might generate enough emotion to produce this same imbalance in mood. In a like manner, many other moods might become fixated by the excessive spread of one or more emotions. Virtually any combination of emotions present in excess might produce a sufficient redistribution of emotional associations to generate a dominant and relatively inflexible mood state. In this way, the various moods characteristic of depression and mania may arise.

CHANGES IN MEMORY STRENGTH IN DEPRESSION AND MANIA

As indicated in this chapter, the redistribution of emotional associations may be a central factor in the development of depression and mania. But such changes probably do not occur without corresponding alterations in the strength of the memories involved. This would seem to be a natural consequence of the proposed interdependence between memories and emotions. Such changes in synaptic conductance may also contribute to the development and maintenance of mood disorders, as will be discussed.

As proposed here, the release of emotion during stimulating situations may drive memory consolidation via the hippocampus. Through repetitive activation, the synaptic junctions within the new memory may gain strength and become more capable of energy conductance. In effect, the path of neurotransmission defining the new structure may become more coherent and distinctive, as compared with other overlapping memory tracts utilizing the same neurons. Such synaptic changes should occur every time a new memory associated with emotion is stored. It should also occur when the emotional component of an established memory changes, as occurs during polarization. This may be particularly relevant during the generation of mood disorders.

The initial increases in synaptic strength and conductance that occur when a new memory is stored or an old memory acquires polarized emotion probably account for the ease of recall exhibited by most fresh memories. This phenomenon was described in the chapter on localization. It was pointed out that memories, such as those of the "reverend," remain fresh and easily retrievable, with minimum cuing, for some time after storage. Over time, more cues may be required for full recall as the original memory undergoes decay. It is presumed here that this decline in memory retention occurs through a partial reversal in the initial synaptic strength produced during storage. Perhaps when the original emotion has dissipated sufficiently to terminate the hippocampal drive, some natural decay in the synaptic structure occurs if repeated stimulation of the memory does not occur. A theoretical basis for these effects is presented in the next few paragraphs.

LONG-TERM POTENTIATION

In the first chapter, the process of *long-term potentiation* (LTP), as originally observed by Bliss and colleagues, was described. This term refers to the increase in synaptic strength that occurs when a brief stimulating current is applied to an afferent nerve fiber. This work, along with later research, has provided direct confirmation for Hebb's original postulate. Perhaps the principles that underlie LTP are the same as those involved in memory storage and the synaptic changes that are postulated to initially occur. The kinetics of LTP certainly appear compatible with this idea. LTP can be produced by brief episodes of electrical activity (Diamond, Dunwiddie, & Ross, 1988); is enhanced by repeated stimulation (Bliss & Lomo, 1973); and decays over time, in the absence of additional stimulation (Barnes, 1979; Racine, Milgram, & Hafner, 1983). These data suggest that some naturally occurring process, similar to LTP, may underlie normal memory storage and influence the strength of the resulting memory structures over time.

It is worth noting at this point that a neural mechanism has been experimentally observed that reverses the increase in synaptic strength produced by LTP (Desmond & Levy, 1983; Stanton & Sejnowski, 1989). It has been proposed that this phenomenon, termed long-term depression, may play a role in the process of forgetting by ridding the brain of trivial information established through LTP (Churchland & Sejnowski, 1992). Obviously, such a mechanism may play a role in the consolidation of generalized memory complexes, and may also contribute to the forgetting produced by retroactive and proactive inhibition.

Emotionally stimulating events are commonplace in life. The ideas presented here suggest that each such occurrence may produce an increase in conductance among the neurons encoding the memory of the event. It was previously suggested that the strength of such a structure may be proportional to the intensity of emotion generated. This, of course, may be directly related to the amount of hippocampal drive received by the new structure during the process of consolidation. As indicated before, such a system would ensure that important events, as designated by strong emotion, would produce durable memories, which would remain available for future reference.

LOCALIZATION AS A FUNCTION OF MEMORY STRENGTH

The strength of a memory may influence its ease of recall. As illustrated in a previous chapter, strong memories appear to require fewer localization cues for retrieval than those that are weaker or older. It is obviously easier to recall a routine event that occurred yesterday than a similar event from 3 months ago. The retrieval of such an older memory might be possible if further information specifying the time, place, and general circumstances of the situation in question were also available. In other words, additional localization cues would be necessary for full recall. In contrast, a strong memory from 3 months ago may require only minimal prompting for full recall. The dependence of retrieval on memory strength seems obvious. Once again, such an arrangement would provide a biological advantage for the brain, in that significant memories would have more access to consciousness than those with less meaning.

The ideas presented here suggest that the associations composing a young, strong memory would be joined by synaptic linkages with enhanced electrical conductance. This might be viewed biochemically as an increase in the amount of neurotransmitter released by presynaptic neurons, or perhaps by a change in receptor number or sensitivity at the postsynaptic terminus. Work with the marine snail *Aplysia* (as described by Kandel and Hawkins in 1992) has demonstrated that there is an increase in the amount of neurotransmitter released as a consequence of classical conditioning (associative learning). In addition, some forms of nonassociative learning (learning that occurs through repetition of a single stimulus rather than the pairing of two or more stimuli) have also been shown to be mediated by increases in neurotransmitter release (Castellucci & Kandel, 1976). Obviously a number of factors, which may include an increase in the amount of neurotransmitter released from presynaptic neurons, may operate at a molecular level to influence synaptic conductance or resistance to ion flow. Regardless of the exact mechanism involved, neurotransmission arriving at a strong memory during the localization process would meet with entities displaying lower intermemory resistance or enhanced energy flow, as compared with structures with lesser degrees of conductance. Energy reaching and activating a single component association of such a strong memory would, in turn, be transmitted easily to the other associations of the parent structure. In contrast, the transmission of energy within a memory with a lower degree of synaptic conduction would reach and activate fewer component associations. In effect, such an arrangement should produce preferential activation of stronger memories. Perhaps this explains why fewer cues would be needed to fully trigger memories with enhanced synaptic conductance.

EMOTIONAL STIMULATION IN MOOD DISORDERS

Depression and mania may each start with events that are emotionally stimulating. Through hippocampal drive, the memories of such events would acquire strength through enhanced conductance. If other events in life produced a balanced variety of emotion, emotional dilution might occur, and hippocampal activity would eventually cease. The original stimulating memories might then begin to experience some fading and loss of overall synaptic conductance. The development of depression or mania would be averted. If the overall prevailing emotional tone were similar to that of the memory undergoing consolidation, emotional dilution might be slowed and hippocampal activity would continue for a longer time. As a consequence, the memories in question would become even stronger and their recall into consciousness would be enhanced, as explained. Under these conditions, the original stimulating event would thus linger in active awareness longer than under other circumstances. Such memories would continue to influence the mood by release of emotion, as long as these conditions existed. The development of depression or mania would be favored.

It is not uncommon for negative events to be so emotionally disruptive as to produce memories that remain in consciousness for prolonged periods of time. In effect, such memories may seem to become fixated in awareness, producing a great deal of rumination and anxiety. Such a situation may produce a mental status that closely resembles depression. In other words, the patient may look, act, and feel depressed, although his or her emotional status at this time might best be described as an adjustment reaction to the situation. At this point, the focus of the dysphoric mood would clearly be the preceding negative events. Although depressive symptoms would be present, true depression would not exist at this point. If such a condition continued for a prolonged time, transfer of negative emotion to other memories might occur, as described previously. As a result, memories other than those of the original precipitating events would be capable of generating the negative mood state. At this juncture, true depression would start. Patients might report a pervasive negative mood, without a clear precipitating focus. In other words, the symptoms of depression would be present, but patients would be unable to relate their feelings to events from experience. They might state that they feel bad all the time but cannot explain why. They might complain that things upset them without apparent reason. The inability to relate dysphoric symptoms to a definable origin in experience often seems to be characteristic of true depression. This condition may develop when emotion associated with negative life events is not effectively diluted and spreads to other memories only peripherally related to the original stimuli.

The ideas presented suggest that memories acquiring transferred polarized emotion during the evolution of depression and mania may subsequently experience an increase in strength. In other words, a change in the pattern of associated emotions may stimulate new hippocampal activity, producing reinforcement of the memory structures involved. As indicated before, an increase in memory conductance should allow such entities to be triggered into consciousness with fewer cues. As a consequence, such memories would be recalled more frequently, which might disproportionately color the mood with emotion consistent with depression or mania. In this way, changes in memory strength might further perpetuate the moods characteristic of these illnesses. It is therefore proposed that the fixed mood states that seem characteristic of mood disorders arise both from emotional polarization and the strengthening of those memories that associate with such emotion. Both processes would act in unison to maintain a relatively fixed state of mood.

It has been postulated that the emotion associated with memories may become skewed or reordered to reflect a single grouping of emotions through the polarization process. As a consequence, new hippocampal activity may be initiated, strengthening those memories that received polarized emotion. Over time, it is conceivable that this pool of strengthened memories may grow quiet large and involve many memories in current usage, to one degree or another. Under these conditions, the mood state characteristic of the polarized emotion may be predominant in consciousness. Memories strengthened in this way may be very easy to recall, thus perpetuating the mood state. Many cues arising from sensory perception or during thought would preferentially activate those memories involved in the polarization process. Under other conditions, such cues might activate any number of memories to which their matching GMCs corresponded. In a state of emotional polarization, there would be a selective activation of those memories that acquired new emotion and were strengthened through renewed hippocampal activity.

Such a state may approximate a closed system, in that a grouping of reinforced memories may serve to perpetuate the polarized mood through their activation. Once neurotransmission entered this complex of strengthened memories, escape would be difficult. In effect, a state of mental fixation would have been established. Thought might be dominated with such memories, and the mood would be perpetuated. It is reasonable to assume that depression and mania may be initiated and maintained by such conditions.

KINDLING

There is another well-known mental phenomenon that may also depend upon a grouping of strengthened neural circuits for its function. If a brief pulse of electrical energy, at a level below that required to produce convulsions, is applied to the brain of an animal, no seizure will result. If this is repeated daily, the seizure threshold will progressively decrease, and eventually the animal will develop a seizure in response to the same level of applied current. Over time, such an animal will generally develop spontaneous seizures, which require no externally applied energy. This progression to active convulsions has been termed kindling.

We can speculate that kindling may be generated in much the same way as long-term potentiation (LTP), discussed earlier. The application of current, in both cases, may increase the electrical conductance of those axons and dendrites through which energy passes. Each successive bolus of current in the kindling process may open new synaptic linkages, promoting increased overall conductance and a wider flow of energy. Eventually, many neural pathways may be recruited, resulting in large, branched networks of cells connected by highly conductive linkages. Like a fresh memory, neurotransmission or current introduced into such a system would be rapidly transmitted throughout its full extent with little resistance. When such a system grew large enough, the activation of a sufficient number of motor neurons would result in an observable seizure. It is also significant that kindling can produce the same changes in microstructure that result when an animal is maintained in an enriched environment, as discussed earlier. Over time, the growth of new axons and dendrites can be observed. Kindling has obvious similarities with those cellular and synaptic changes that are thought to mediate new learning.

In the process of learning, the natural flow of neurotransmission into neural structures during the matching and localization process may initially produce LTP. A repetition of this process over time may result in the growth of new cellular projections, thus consolidating the memories in question. In kindling, the application of an exogenous current to an animal's brain may produce the same changes in neural architecture. Very large networks of electrically connected neurons may be established in much the same way as large memories. Unlike the learning process, the networks generated through kindling would involve vastly more neurons than even the largest memories and, of course, would not encode meaningful information. The stimulation of a portion of such a complex may produce its activation as a whole, in much the same way as a large, fresh memory is triggered into consciousness. Rather than memory recall, a convulsive episode would result.

KINDLING AS A MODEL FOR BIPOLAR MOOD DISORDER

The kindling phenomenon has been used by others as a model for the spontaneous changes that occur over time in the course of bipolar mood disorder (BMD), as well as recurrent depression. Such changes may take several forms. As the illness progresses, the time course usually becomes accelerated. Transitions from one phase of the illness to next may become more rapid, and the interim periods of relative healthiness may shorten. Response to drug therapy may show corresponding alterations. A patient who is well controlled on one drug for many years may gradually become unresponsive. This may be especially true if the medication is stopped and reinstated at a later time. Other spontaneous changes can also be observed in most patients. Precipitating psychosocial or physical stressors can usually be identified in initial episodes of depression or mania. This identification may become increasingly more difficult with each successive episode of illness. In some way, the illness seems to become more autonomous and less dependent upon external factors. This observation was first made by the German psychiatrist, Emil Kraepelin, in the early part of this century and has been subsequently reported by others (Angst, 1966; Dunner, Murphy, Stallone, & Fieve, 1979). Like kindling, the natural course of BMD seems to progress over time in a spontaneous manner. For an excellent discussion of this subject, see Post (1993).

ANTICONVULSANTS AND BIPOLAR MOOD DISORDER

Because of the similarities described earlier, drugs that are known to control seizures have been tried in patients with BMD. In at least two cases, amazing results have been observed. Both carbamazepine and valproic acid, which are two commonly used anticonvulsants, have also proven to be highly effective in the treatment of BMD. Both medications are now widely used as mood stabilizers in this psychiatric condition. This observation suggests that the similarities between affective disorders and seizures may be more than coincidental. Perhaps both conditions arise from extensively interconnected networks of neural pathways, as proposed here. In some way, both drugs may prevent the full expression of such circuitry, producing symptomatic improvement in these disorders.

ELECTROCONVULSIVE THERAPY

There is at least one more piece of evidence that supports the proposed relationship between seizure disorders and BMD. Electroconvulsive therapy (ECT, or shock treatment) has long been recognized as a rapid and highly effective therapy for depression. ECT is also a very effective treatment of mania (Black, Winokur, & Nasrallah, 1987; Small et al., 1988), but it is rarely used today because of the availability of effective medication. If BMD and seizures both have a similar neural basis, ECT should also alter the course of convulsions. This is exactly what is often seen in clinical settings. Surprisingly, ECT has been shown to have anticonvulsive properties. Repeated shock therapy is known to raise the seizure threshold and decrease the duration of induced seizures. In addition, kindling can be effectively blocked by the administration of ECT (Kellner, 1993).

It has been postulated here that the type of seizures originating from experimental kindling may arise from a large complex of neurons, which are extensively and randomly connected with highly conductive synaptic linkages. It has been suggested that such a complex may be activated as a whole in much the same way as a large, fresh memory. BMD has been characterized as arising from nonrandom neural complexes of memories, which are also strong and highly conductive. This grouping of memories would also constitute a single, electrically coupled complex, because its component entities would all be linked to the same, common set of emotional associations. Both situations are similar, in that each seems to involve patterns of electrically coupled neurons from which neurotransmission cannot easily escape. ECT may be beneficial for both conditions by breaking up or fragmenting the underlying neural patterns that allow each disorder to be maintained and expressed. By forcing current through such pathological circuits, many new routes of neurotransmission may be established and the original neural organization destroyed.

THE ACCELERATION OF MOOD DISORDERS OVER TIME

The tendency for bipolar mood disorder or recurrent depression to accelerate in course over time was discussed previously. Obviously there may be many reasons for this. Perhaps recurrent mood disorders become more autonomous if recovery from successive episodes does not occur fully. In other words, some residue of polarized emotion may remain associated with a small percentage of memories, even after clinical recovery appears complete. Such emotion may not significantly alter the current mood but may provide a starting point for subsequent episodes. For example, psychosocial stressors that trigger memories with residual emotion from a prior episode may be perceived differently because of the residual effects of an earlier illness. In just the right circumstances, this might be sufficient for the initiation of a new episode. After several such recurrences of illness, relatively small life stressors might be sufficient to trigger additional episodes because of an accumulation of lasting polarized emotion. In effect, the illness may become more autonomous over time and less dependent upon life stressors for initiation.

THE DISTRIBUTION OF EMOTIONAL ASSOCIATIONS

It has been proposed that thoughts traveling through consciousness acquire emotion from the prevailing mood. From ideas presented previously, we can predict that this process is probably not random but may be guided by natural lines of association. In other words, the associations of a memory may determine the type and quantity of emotion it acquires. As a consequence, emotion may not be equally distributed to all memories passing through consciousness. Some memories may associate with higher levels of emotion than others, depending on their sequence in thought. This may be an important concept, and it is based upon the following reasoning.

It has been suggested that when memories of stimulating events are considered in consciousness, emotion is released into the prevailing mood. From general observation, such emotion seems to gradually fade over time if the associated memory is not continually stimulated. As a consequence, thoughts that pass through consciousness shortly after the release of such emotion should be exposed to higher emotional levels than those at later times. For example, a thought cycling through the brain 3 minutes after strong emotional release should be exposed to higher emotional levels in the mood than one entering awareness after 10 minutes. Such an arrangement should influence the intensity of emotion that associates with the cycling thought. We can therefore predict that some memories may acquire more emotion from the mood than others because of this differential level of exposure that each should experience.

It has also been proposed that each new thought passing through consciousness is constructed from memories associated with those used to compose previous thoughts. In other words, the associations triggered by a given thought on its passage through the brain will provide the raw material for the next thought in the sequence. One association leads to the next, and so forth, often resulting in long chains of interconnected mental activity. As indicated earlier, this probably explains why thinking is normally coherent and associated in nature. Because of this arrangement, each thought occurring in sequence would be closely related through association to the one that just preceded it. As such a chain grew, each successive thought generated would be less well associated with the first entity of the sequence. In other words, the farther two items were from each other in such a series, the less associative relationship they would have. This would seem to be a natural consequence of a system based upon associated memories.

These ideas suggest that the transfer of emotion in consciousness is most likely to occur between memories that are the most closely related through association. This would seem to be true, because emotion added to the mood during the interpretation of a thought would be at its maximum intensity during those times when the most highly associated memories were passing though consciousness. Over time, such emotion would progressively fade from the mood and form weaker associations with subsequent thoughts, which would also be less well associated with the original source of emotion. In other words, the rate of decay experienced by an emotion in the mood should generally parallel the progressive decrease in associative relationship between the original source of emotion and each subsequent entity that passes through the brain. As a result of this theoretical arrangement, it is likely that emotion would be most readily transferred to those thoughts with the greatest natural associative relationship to the original thought that produced the emotion.

When neural structures that encode memory and emotion are localized and activated during cyclic thought, perceptions arise that are sensed consciously. It has been proposed that when such entities enter active awareness in close succession, strong associative relationships are formed between them. In contrast, entities arriving in consciousness, separated by greater intervals of time, form correspondingly weaker associative relationships. In other words, the degree of association that results between emotions and memories entering consciousness may, in most cases, be a function of their temporal proximities. In some ways, these ideas are conceptually consistent with the tenets of classical conditioning (associative learning), as originally stated by Pavlov (1927) in his book entitled Conditioned Reflexes. When stimuli to be paired are presented at intervals from a fraction of a second to a few seconds, strong associative relationships are produced. As these time intervals are increased, progressively weaker pairings are observed, as indicated by a reduced ability of conditioned stimuli to produce conditioned responses. It is therefore suggested that the associative relationships that are established when thoughts and emotions pass through consciousness may constitute a form of classical conditioning.

As discussed earlier in this chapter, strong emotion that lingers in consciousness for prolonged periods of time may not be subject to the same temporal limitations that seem to apply in classical conditioning. In such cases, intense emotion, which is deposited in the mood, may remain viable for long periods of time and be capable of associating with thoughts that enter consciousness at much later times. In other words, the time restrictions of classical conditioning may not be as important in such situations as the intensity of the emotion that endures in consciousness. In the majority of cases, emotion released into the mood during interpretation of data probably dissipates rapidly, producing little, if any, association with temporally distant thoughts passing through consciousness. The formation of associative relationships may therefore be subject to the tenets of classical conditioning under most normal conditions of mood. On occasion, emotion arising from intensely stimulating events may not dissipate as rapidly, and may remain in the mood for extended periods of times. Under such conditions, a disproportionate spread of emotion to many more memories than normal may occur, and depression or mania may ultimately result.

The ideas expressed here suggest that the transfer of emotion, which is postulated to be a function of consciousness, is not random but may follow lines of association dictated by the natural organization of memories. In other words, the transfer of emotion is probably most efficient between those memories with close, natural, associative relationships, for the reasons described. Such an arrangement predicts that all thoughts passing through consciousness would not acquire emotion equally. The degree of emotional association that resulted would largely be a function of the natural relationship between memories composing the thought and those serving as the source of the emotion. The nonrandom nature of this process may help explain certain aspects of mood disorders that have long been clinically observed.

It has been postulated that depression and mania evolve when intense emotion becomes redistributed to many memories in current usage. The ideas presented in the last few paragraphs suggests that this spread of emotion may follow lines of association. The first memories to become involved in the polarization process would be those with the highest natural degree of association with the central memories of the stimulating events. Such closely associated memories would, of course, be the most likely to be considered in thought immediately following recall of the original stimulating issues. Over time, emotion would gradually spread to less well-associated memories that entered consciousness. Eventually, some memories with only distant relationships to the principle issues might become involved. In effect, emotional transfer would follow established associative gradients.

It seems probable that the spreading process would be driven by the intensity of central emotion arising from the original stimulating events. Such emotion may gradually migrate outward from its original source, along lines of association, to affect many secondary memories. The extent of spread would ultimately be a function of the overall amount of emotional dilution encountered. We can speculate that the original migrating emotion would blend with the associated emotion linked with each memory encountered along the associative pathway and, as a result, would experience some dilution. Eventually the spreading process would halt, when the original emotion was sufficiently dissipated.

The development of an episode of mood disorder might occur when the intense emotion associated with a central core of memories spread outward, involving many less directly related memories. As indicated before, this process would largely be nonrandom, in that the most likely memories to acquire emotion would be those with some degree of natural association with the original central issues. Completely unrelated memories would acquire little, if any, transferred emotion. Such memories would simply not be triggered into consciousness with any significant frequency during times when the stimulating events were being considered and emotion was being transferred.

ISOLATED POCKETS OF POLARIZED EMOTION

These ideas suggest that mood disorders may result from the growth of relatively isolated pockets of associated memories linked to a single blend of intense emotion. Once neurotransmission entered such an area, escape might be difficult because of the increased electrical conductance of the involved neural circuitry. As discussed before, this may be a consequence of memories associated with intense emotion. Under these conditions, there would literally be a mental preoccupation with the involved memories, and the mood would be perpetuated in consciousness. The greater the spread of involved emotion, the more difficult escape would become, and the more entrenched would be the mood disorder. Through this sequence of events, the fixed mood states characteristic of these disorders may evolve.

It has been postulated that the transfer of emotion in consciousness follows lines of association, because thought itself is governed by such relationships. The spread of a single blend of emotion to many memories may occur when a situation encoded in memory is intense and cannot be adequately dealt with through emotional dilution. Through lines of association, many individual memories may acquire a similar blend of emotion, and eventually large isolated complexes may develop. Because of the nonrandom nature of this process, other unassociated brain regions may remain relatively normal and unaffected by this process of polarization. These concepts may help to explain several clinical observations associated with affective disorders, as will be discussed.

MOOD SWINGS

Mood lability is a common feature in depression and mania. This symptom is especially noticeable in the early stages of these disorders, when rapid shifts in emotional status may occur frequently in response to relatively minor environmental or mental events. In many cases, there may be no recognizable precipitating factor. Patients usually report dramatic and unexpected changes in their prevailing mood, which may be very distressing. Such mood swings often signal the onset of more severe illness.

The ideas presented suggest that this form of mood instability may be a direct consequence of the pockets, or zones, of intense emotion that may result from polarization. According to this theoretical arrangement, clusters of associated memories, linked to a single blending of emotion, may accumulate as a mood disorder evolves. Thought originating from memories outside such a complex might be relatively free of this intense emotion, and be generally normal in content. When a memory from within such a complex is localized and activated by a random thought or environmental stimuli, intense emotion may be released, producing a rapid change in the predominant mental state. The mood swing would be easily perceived because of the large contrast it produced in the existing emotional tone of the patient. In the absence of such pockets of intensely polarized emotion, changes in mood can certainly occur but are generally not as rapid or intense. It is certainly possible that some degree of polarization is normally present within the brain, allowing small shifts in mood to be perceived. The extreme mood swings seen in pathological conditions may be the direct consequence of the excessive segregation of memories produced when emotional associations become extensively skewed.

AREAS OF OPPOSING EMOTIONAL POLARIZATION

In the early stages of mood disorders, patients often display intense levels of emotion that seem to be driven by enhanced mood lability. This disruption in mental status may initially be mild and appear only as an increase in irritability, accompanied by moodiness. Such changes may, however, be the consequences of early polarization. As emotional redistribution continues, groups of memories might become more segregated and, as a consequence, mood swings might become more prominent and noticeable. Because the process of emotional polarization may selectively follow lines of association, many unrelated memories in storage may not be affected by this process. This, of course, would not be true if polarization were a random process affecting all memories equally. Because of this theoretical arrangement, it is possible that isolated pockets of emotion might arise simultaneously with similar or even opposing emotional blends. This would seem possible if a variety of emotionally contrasting life events occurred, involving memories with little prior association. Under these conditions, pockets of dysphoric emotion might simultaneously develop and coexist in relative isolation with areas of intense positive or energizing emotion. This concept is illustrated in Figure 8.5.

MIXED STATES

The clinical picture produced when opposing emotion becomes polarized within the same general time frame may be responsible for the generation of the mixed state. This condition is well known in psychiatry and often precedes the onset of more serious illness. It is characterized by extreme mood lability, producing elements of both depression and mania. A patient may display manic-like symptoms that alternate with

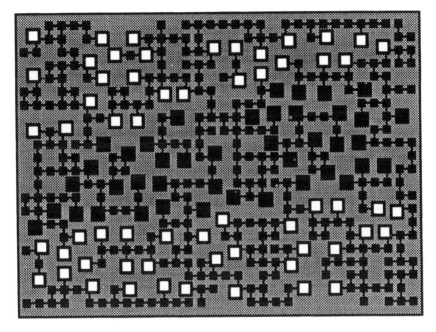

Figure 8.5 The concept of "polarized zones of emotion" is illustrated here. Small, black squares represent neurons, and the larger black-and-white squares indicate associated emotion, which is opposite in type. Note that the zone of "black" emotion in the middle of the figure is surrounded by areas of "white" emotion. Such zones of polarization may explain many of the symptoms of mood disorders, as explained in the text. It is important to note that such zones probably do not exist within the brain as physically isolated groupings of emotion, as depicted in this figure. This is done here only for the purpose of illustration. Within the brain, such zones probably exist as electrical, coherent networks joining component entities, which may be widely separated in three-dimensional space.

those typical of depression. A common clinical picture may include racing thoughts, suicidal ideation, auditory hallucinations, persecutory delusions, insomnia, agitation, and hypersexuality, framed by alternating moods that may be elevated and euphoric at some times and dysphoric at others (Akiskal, 1983; Himmelhoch, Mulla, Neil, Detre, & Kupfer, 1976). A chaotic mixture of opposing emotions may be displayed in relatively short periods of time. It is conceivable that such a situation might be produced by thought moving through polarized zones of intense and opposing emotion. In other words, such a state may originate from the same conditions that produce mood swings.

Mixed states are common in bipolar mood disorder. In their 1990 book entitled Manic–Depressive Illness, Goodwin and Jamison have summarized data from eight studies, utilizing a total of 506 bipolar patients, and have concluded that an average of 40.1% of such cases displayed mixed states. The range between individual studies was large (16–67%), which probably reflects differences in inclusion criteria. Obviously this condition is far from rare.

Mixed states often precede episodes of full-blown mania or depression. This is consistent with the idea that mood instability is at least partially the product of emotional polarization. As a mood disorder progresses, polarization in one or more clusters of memories may spread. As a consequence, one or more mood states may eventually become dominant. It also seems possible that several polarized clusters of memories with similar emotion may coalesce to generate a large grouping of memories that may dominate consciousness by producing a fixed and largely inescapable mood state.

RAPID CYCLING

In some rare cases, it is conceivable that the extensive spread of opposing, polarized emotion in different groupings of memories may occur simultaneously. Eventually, two or more large, separate emotional domains may evolve. Under these conditions, no single emotional complex may be capable of completely dominating consciousness for extended periods of time. When a transition from one domain to the next occurs, a dramatic shift from one mood state to another would be experienced. Such a situation may provide a theoretical basis for the rapid cycling exhibited by a small percentage of patients (13–20% per Goodwin and Jamison, 1990) with bipolar mood disorder. Although rapid cycling is usually defined as four or more affective episodes per year, cycles as short as 48 (ultrarapid cyclers) have been observed. The ideas proposed here suggest that rapid shifts from profound depression to mania, or vice versa, may be possible because of the simultaneous existence of emotional domains of opposing content.

The theory presented here suggests that mood swings, mixed states, and rapid cycling may all arise from the same basic conditions that give rise to mood disorders themselves. When polarization is moderate, mood swings may be prominent. When some degree of opposing emotion becomes polarized, drastic shifts in mood states may occur, producing mixed states. If a given emotional type becomes dominant, a full-blown episode of mania or depression may appear. In rare cases, extensive areas of opposing emotion may be present, and shifts in mood may produce the phenomenon of rapid cycling. Obviously, many biological and environmental factors may influence the evolution of illness in such a complex system.

DELUSIONS IN MOOD DISORDERS

In both depression and mania, psychosis is common. Patients with either disorder frequently display delusional thought content or experience hallucinations (Black & Nasrallah, 1989; Rosenthal, Rosenthal, Stallone, Dunner, & Fieve, 1980; Winokur et al., 1969). The ideas presented in subsequent paragraphs represent an attempt to provide a rational, theoretical explanation for such symptoms. It is proposed that a failure to appreciate reality may be directly related to a decrease in the number of moods available to these patients. Under such conditions, state-dependent memory effects may become excessive and produce symptoms of psychosis.

Emotions seem to act as labels that become associated with the events of our lives as they are recorded in memory. They provide the brain with an understanding of the type and degree of significance attached to each event we experience. When a memory is triggered into consciousness, its associated emotional component reproduces the interpretation of the original event, and emotion from the mood blends with it to provide current relevancy. This was discussed in a previous chapter. In most cases, emotion from the mood probably updates the retrieved memory but may not extensively alter its original interpretation. Under most conditions, this probably provides a reasonably accurate assessment of the current situation. At other times, emotion derived from an intense mood might be much stronger than that from the reference memory. On these occasions, the dominant tone might unduly influence the overall interpretation of the original memory. As a consequence, the events under current consideration may show some mild and transient deviation from reality.

Such mild distortions in thinking are probably commonplace in daily life. Many examples can be cited. A minor inconvenience might be seen as major, or a casual acquaintance might be greeted with the same enthusiasm as an old friend. In almost any situation, we may react in an inappropriate manner if there is sufficient emotional bias from the dominant mood. Pleasurable events, as well as those of a more dysphoric nature, may experience some degree of distortion under conditions of intense mood. Such mild interpretive errors can often be seen in the judgments we make. A predominant mood of optimism and carefree feelings might blend with the anticipation of owning a new car to cause us to make a purchase we could not really afford. In other cases, our decisions may be more conservative than necessary because of a mood of excessive cautiousness. Interpretative distortions such as these are common and probably unavoidable. Such errors are often recognized in quieter, more reflective moments. They may have few long-term consequences when a balanced array of moods is available for mental reference. In pathological states, where the number of available mood states may be limited, the cumulative effects of such errors may be much more significant. Such minor distortions in thought may produce delusions and other symptoms of frank psychosis.

The prolonged, negative mood characteristic of depression may generate many minor distortions in thought, which may accumulate and become noticeable over time. These patients may worry excessively about trivial things and generally show emotional reactions that are not in proportion to the events occurring. For example, a patient may ruminate for an hour about spilling a glass of milk. It may be perceived as a major tragedy and produce a greatly exaggerated sense of guilt. Obviously this emotional interpretation of the event is flawed and may even have a delusional flavor. Other patients may misinterpret a simple act of kindness by a family member as having a hidden, sinister meaning. Paranoia may even develop as a cognitive response to the situation. Patients may even come to fear that their food is poisoned or that others are plotting to kill them. They might even view certain of their own frightening thoughts as being alien and originating from an outside source. Auditory hallucinations are not unusual in severe depression. It is conceivable that an extensive degree of negative emotional association might cause these distortions in reality. These effects are common in depression, where an intense, abnormal mood may persist for long periods of time. When the mood returns to normal, these minor deviations in thought, as well as symptoms that are frankly psychotic, spontaneously remit.

Perhaps a hypothetical example might help to understand the process by which psychosis might develop. Assume that a severely depressed man is admitted to the hospital for treatment. His mood is predominantly negative and consists largely of anxiety, fear, and sadness. As with most patients, he is placed on a regular diet, and his tray of food is delivered three times a day. Mealtime is normally pleasurable for him, although his interest in eating may have diminished somewhat lately. Each time a tray of food is delivered to him, it triggers his general memories of eating, as well as its emotional component. On each such occasion, the memory of this normally pleasurable event blends with his dysphoric mood, producing a small amount of negative association, which is stored with the memory. Eventually, eating may become perceived as an unpleasant or even fearful event as negative emotion accumulates with the involved memories. He may come to dread mealtime for reasons that are not completely clear to him. In an attempt to understand his fears, he may assume the food is poisoned. Reasoning such as this would provide him with a logical explanation for his fears. Of course, he may fixate on any number of possible explanations for his unexplained emotions. He may come to feel that the nurse who brings him his tray is trying to kill him, or that another patient may use his dinner knife to stab him. His content of thought may take any form and is not the driving force in the delusion. It is simply the focus of thought that makes the most sense to him at the time. It is his best explanation for the feelings he is experiencing. The mismatch in emotion is the driving force behind his delusion. Their negative nature supports the delusional thoughts, making them seem plausible. In a nondepressed person, thoughts such as these would be dismissed as foolish. There would be no emotional support for them. In depression, the inappropriate spread of negative emotion on a grand scale may allow patients to fixate on thoughts that seem to justify their feelings. Through this process, bizarre ideas may take on a sense of realism because of erroneous emotional support.

A careful observer in the right circumstances can often see the progression of a delusion in a depressed patient. Initially, there may be some guarded comments about a troubling thought. For example, a female patient may tell you that she fears her son is dead. Careful questioning may reveal that there is no rationale for this conclusion. At this point, the thought may be more speculation than delusion. Over time, the thought may become more fixed, and the patient may be more sure of its truthfulness, despite a complete lack of objective evidence. When asked to justify her belief, she probably can give no logical explanation. She may only comment that she feels that he is dead. In other words, proof to her is solely emotional in nature and may be completely unshaken by facts to the contrary. Even if her son suddenly appeared, she might not believe it was him. He might be viewed as an impostor or perhaps even the spirit of her son. These might be considered rational explanations, considering her emotional bias. In this example, the influence of emotion on thought is obvious. The psychotic part of this process seems driven by the distorted emotional tone rather than the cognitive conclusions themselves. Such thoughts may be relatively normal, given the extreme degree of emotional disturbance present.

As suggested, distortions in normal thought may arise when an emotional tone is dominant and excessively influences interpretations arising from retrieved memories. We are probably all subject to this at one time or another. This effect seems directly attributable to the bias imposed by a strong prevailing mood state. At later times, when different moods are present, such distortions may be realized. Alternate moods may provide access to different memories, which allow the original situation to be viewed in a truer, more balanced light. In effect, the availability of other moods provides us with a greater cognitive perspective. Under normal mood conditions, such minor distortions in thought eventually become corrected. In pathological states, the number of moods available may be greatly restricted. Partial or complete amnesia for memories associated with other moods may exist. In effect, important information, which is normally available for reference, may be absent. Under these conditions, the distortions that arise from biased mood states may not be corrected. False beliefs may persist and grow in the absence of balancing information. Things normally recognized as being incorrect or even ridiculous may seem perfectly reasonable in the absence of contradicting data. This seems to be a reasonably simple explanation for the delusional psychosis often seen in mood disorders.

AUDITORY HALLUCINATIONS IN MOOD DISORDERS

The ideas expressed here seem to provide a rational explanation for the delusions that frequently occur in depression and mania. Auditory hallucinations are a second form of psychosis common to these disorders. As postulated in the previous chapter, the hallucinations of MPD may result from the isolated mood conditions that underlie this disorder. Verbal thoughts arising in one personality domain may appear alien when perceived by a second personality structure lacking the memories necessary for full interpretation. In these cases, it is not surprising that such thoughts are often perceived as voices originating from some mysterious outside source. The mechanism driving this process may also produce the auditory hallucinations seen in depression and mania.

In MPD, it is postulated that isolated pockets of memories originate and grow in association with specific emotional entities. This process may generate the conditions necessary for the production of auditory hallucinations, as discussed previously. In patients without MPD, such isolated conditions probably do not exist to any significant extent. Memories may be normally blended with each other through the sharing of common emotional associations, as described in the previous chapter. It is postulated here that this normal level of integration may break down when emotional associations become skewed or polarized during the evolution of mood disorders.

Most memories are probably associated with a number of different emotions, which collectively define their meaning within the brain. Such memories may be extensively integrated with many others through the sharing of these common emotions. Through polarization, the diversity of such associations may eventually become narrowed. Under such conditions, the segregation of memories into isolated aggregates might eventually occur if polarization were extensive. As indicated before, this is probably basic to the evolution of mood disorders. Once such complexes became fully established, relatively fixed mood states would dominate. Under these conditions, the escape of conscious thought from such a complex might be difficult because of the intense emotion present and the increase in synaptic conductance that would result. At this point, a situation similar to that seen in MPD might exist. Segregated groupings of memories, each capable of some degree of independent data interpretation, would provide a potential for psychotic thought. It is therefore proposed that the auditory hallucinations of depression and mania may arise from the same isolated conditions thought to exist in MPD.

PSYCHOTHERAPY

In many cases, psychotherapy is beneficial for patients with depression. Through this process, a skilled therapist can guide and shape patients' cognitive and emotional perception of their illness. Over time, symptomatic improvement will often occur. This process may be a way of progressively altering or diluting negative emotion associated with thought. In other words, the mental changes postulated to occur in depression may be reversed. These ideas will be discussed in the following paragraphs.

When new memories are created, they are exposed to the mood from which they gain an emotional interpretation. In this way, information from matching memories, as well as the prevailing emotional tone, becomes associated and is stored with the new entity. When older memories are recalled, they should also acquire new emotion from the current mood in much the same way. This association would be expected because of the exposure of the activated memory to the dominant mood when they mix in consciousness.

These processes may have important consequences for the brain. If a memory were frequently recalled over time, its original emotional component should become diluted through new association. This concept was introduced earlier in this chapter. Eventually its associated emotion should represent a composite of the various moods to which the recalled memory was exposed. This process would serve to update the interpretation of the memory, allowing it to maintain relevancy. In this way, the emotion associated with a memory may change over time to reflect current issues.

Perhaps an example might help to illustrate this proposed process of emotional dilution. Let us suppose your wedding was a joyful and festive event. Through the years, these memories may be recalled multiple times in various emotional situations. Each time this occurred, some of the current emotional tone would enter association with the original memory. Over time, the joyful emotion that was initially stored would become diluted. Each time the events were recalled, less of this original emotion would be experienced. Eventually, it might be largely replaced with a somewhat neutral emotional component, derived cumulatively through repeated recall and new emotional association. The emotion of the original event might appear faded, although the memory of the wedding itself might be largely intact. Most memories probably lose their dominant emotional component through this dilutional process.

Many people have observed that the emotion associated with memories is frequently lost before the memory itself deteriorates. We often can recall an event occurring years ago, but the emotion experienced at the time of storage can no longer be fully sensed. This is a common experience. In his book entitled The Brain (1984), Richard Restak noted that a photograph of an early childhood event in his life caused memory recall, but the joyful emotion originally experienced could not be retrieved. Most people probably have many such memories, which remain at least partially viable, despite the loss of the emotional component. This could be the direct result of the emotional dilution postulated to occur over time, when a memory is frequently recalled. The original emotional component may not actually be lost, but may become so diluted that it is not easily recognizable.

PROACTIVE INHIBITION AND EMOTIONAL DILUTION

Perhaps emotional dilution might best be characterized as a form of proactive inhibition. This well-established psychological phenomenon refers to the loss in retention experienced by an older memory when new material of a similar nature is stored in memory. In other words, new learning can interfere with the recall of older learning in some circumstances. This concept, as it relates to the forgetting of learned information, was discussed in an earlier chapter. In the present context, each new emotion (new learning) that associates with a memory should produce an increase in competitive interference with older emotions already linked with the memory. As with any association subjected to proactive inhibition, some retention loss would be expected, which should be reflected as a reduction in the perceptual intensity of the original emotion in a situation producing its recall. This, of course, appears to be conceptually identical to the process of emotional dilution, which has been described here. From this perspective, emotional dilution might be viewed as a form of forgetting, not unlike that experienced with other types of stored information.

This type of emotional fading probably occurs with all memories that are used with any frequency. This would seem to be particularly true with GMCs that receive heavy usage. Over time, most memories probably lose their ability to induce perceptible emotion when recalled. In reality, their associated emotion may have become neutral, due to the repeated dilution from frequent recall. Interpretations using these memories are probably less emotional and more literal in nature. In other words, these memories are used to understand events as they literally occur in experience. For example, words used in a conversation might be translated into visual images or other sensory terms to understand some event being described by a speaker. Other sounds or visual data perceived directly would be matched with stored memories, resulting in an understanding of the physical events occurring. Very little, if any, emotional interpretation would result or be necessary for this type of literal translation. Many of our experiences are routine and require no emotional component for full understanding. Presumably, emotion would no longer be necessary for localization of such frequently used memories. In our daily activities, emotional and literal interpretations are probably constantly blended to derive a full understanding of the world around us.

As suggested here, the emotional component of a memory may become diluted by the addition of new emotion derived from the prevailing mood. Because emotions appear to be associations of memories, a second form of emotional dilution would also seem possible. It is conceivable that a new memory added in association with the primary memory might also serve to dilute the original emotional component. Neurotransmission reaching and activating the primary memory would now be transmitted to more associations than before addition of the new memory. The original emotional association would be less strongly activated because of competition with the new association. This would appear to be a variation on the process of proactive interference, which results in the forgetting of memories through associative competition. Because emotion appears to be a form of memory association, it, too, should be subject to some forgetting by the same mechanism. And so, it is proposed that this form of emotional dilution may also occur through competitive interference.

EMOTIONAL DILUTION AS A BASIS FOR PSYCHOTHERAPY

Emotional dilution is probably the basis for psychotherapy. As part of this process, traumatic past events are discussed with a trained therapist in an atmosphere of acceptance and safety. Patients are allowed to confront their problems in a controlled environment, in which there is the expectation of improvement. The same issues may be dealt with in one form or another over several weeks or months. Through this process, many patients learn to cope with memories that have perhaps been painful for years. In this way, the negative emotion seems to lose some of its impact, allowing patients to face the issues more squarely. It seems possible that this occurs through a progressive dilution of the painful emotion associated with the original memories. In effect, the patient is being desensitized by the establishment of new associations that dilute the old. Each time a painful memory is recalled, it acquires a small amount of the prevailing emotional tone. In this way, some of the positive emotion generated by the therapist, as well as the calm, controlled atmosphere of the therapy setting, is transferred to the negative memories under consideration. Despite the many schools and philosophies of psychotherapy, this may be the common thread by which they all produce beneficial results.

SYSTEMATIC DESENSITIZATION

The theoretical basis for psychotherapy suggested here is in general agreement with older ideas. Edwin R. Guthrie (1886–1959) was an early, influential learning theorist, who believed that extinction or forgetting of a memory was always the result of associative competition (Guthrie, 1935). In other words, he believed that if there were no interference from new learning, there would be no forgetting. This, of course, is the theory of proactive and retroactive interference, which was discussed earlier. Using these ideas, he developed a theoretical basis for the breaking of unwanted habits. These ideas were then adopted by many psychotherapists to help their patients overcome debilitating emotional problems and their behavioral consequences. One example of this is systematic desensitization (SD), as popularized by Wolpe in 1958. The negative emotion associated with phobias and other traumatic memories can often be reduced using this technique. It is proposed here that emotional dilution is the underlying mechanism that drives such emotional changes. Perhaps a closer look at SD might provide some insight into the manipulation of emotion by the brain.

It has been postulated that thoughts and perceptions passing through consciousness acquire emotion from the prevailing mood. This basic assumption underlies a number of larger concepts presented in this work. Unfortunately, this associative process is difficult, if not impossible, to observe directly, under most normal conditions of thought. Mental processes simply seem too well integrated and complex for this effect to be detected as an individual entity. SD may, however, provide a unique opportunity to view this process in relative isolation.

As suggested earlier, the basis of SD seems to be emotional dilution. Prior to the initiation of therapy, the patient is extensively interviewed to establish a list of anxiety-producing situations related to the original traumatic events. These items are then ranked in an anxiety hierarchy, based upon the amount of negative emotion evoked by each. On one end of this list are those things that are the least anxiety producing and the most casually related to the disturbing events. The original traumatic situation itself lies at the other extreme of this emotional continuum.

The patient is taught deep-muscle relaxation, and then progressively is exposed to a graded series of imagined situations from the hierarchy list. The process starts with those memories that evoke the least fear and anxiety, followed by those associated with more intense emotion. Through this guided and progressive exposure to fearful thoughts, the patient eventually makes new associations with the pleasant feelings produced by the deep-muscle relaxation and the reassuring atmosphere of the therapeutic environment. In other words, anxiety-producing thoughts appear to acquire new emotion from the nonthreatening mood. Because the fearful situations are slowly presented to the patient in a controlled way, positive associations are formed before any appreciable anxiety can be stimulated. By mastering fears in this stepwise fashion, the patient is able to progressively move to more threatening situations. At each level of the process, new positive associations from the mood are added to dilute the old, fearful emotion. In essence, the patient relearns new emotional responses to old fear-inducing stimuli. Through emotional dilution, negative feelings are gradually weakened through competition with new emotion, and patients eventually

becomes better able to deal with their concerns. Although this is a specific technique, the general principles of emotional dilution probably operate in all forms of talk therapy.

The technique described appears to directly utilize the process of
emotional dilution. At each level of the hierarchy, the small amount of
negative emotion evoked is diluted by opposing emotion from the nonthreatening mood. This presumably reduces the total emotion of the
original situation somewhat, enabling the patient to tolerate the next
level of the hierarchy. Eventually, most, if not all, the original emotion is
neutralized, and thoughts of the phobia or frightening events can be better tolerated. Analysis of this technique allows direct observation of
emotional dilution in an isolated context and seems to provide support
for the contention that memories passing through consciousness acquire
emotion from the prevailing mood.

In the technique of SD, a graded list of anxiety-producing situations
is initially established, as described. Each item on this list is related in
some way to memories of the original traumatic situation. The hypothesis presented here predicts that the degree of similarity between such
items would be a function of the number of shared associations. It seems
reasonable to assume that items evoking strong emotion would share
many common associations with the original situation, whereas those
stimulating weaker emotion would contain only a few. This, of course, is
consistent with the concept of stimulus generalization, which suggests
that the degree of overlap exhibited by memories determines their response to a given stimulus. When an item of low resemblance to the
original situation is imagined by a patient, memories of the original situation would also receive some stimulation in the localization process,
through associations that are common to both structures. Although the
original memory would receive insufficient stimulation for activation as
a whole, it seems reasonable to assume that a small amount of emotion
might be released. This would seem especially true if the original memory were strong and its linkages showed a high degree of electrical conductance, as discussed earlier. As items of greater similarity were considered, the number of shared associations would increase, and the
original memory would experience a greater amount of activation energy. As a consequence, more emotion should be released into consciousness, signifying an increased similarity between the two entities.
At each level of the hierarchy, the emotion triggered by the activation of
common associations would be diluted by contributions from the mood.
The total amount of emotion associated with the original memory
would thus be diminished somewhat at each level, making it possible
for the patient to take the next step without experiencing an increase in

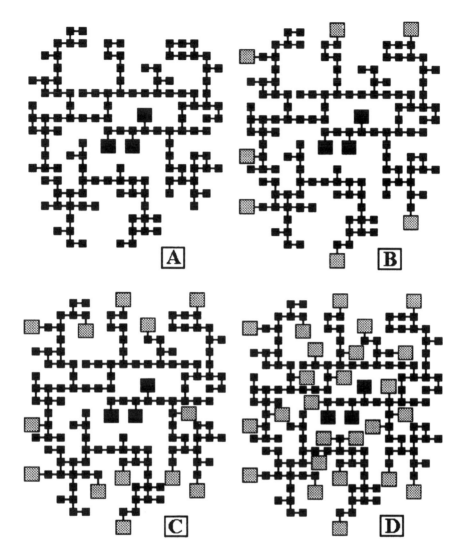

Figure 8.6 The emotional dilution that produces systematic desensitization is illustrated. In Part A of this figure, a grouping of memories encoding a traumatic event is shown. The three large, black squares represent intense, associated negative emotion. Small, black squares represent neurons or groupings of neurons. At the periphery of Structure A are memories that are less well associated with the traumatic event. These are memories that would be the lowest on the anxiety-hierarchy scale and would evoke the least amount of negative emotion on recall. The most highly associated memories are located near the center of the structure. Activation of these memories would stimulate the most intense, negative emotion. As the process of systematic desensitization proceeds, positive emotion is added from the periphery inward, as shown in Parts B–D. Gray squares represent various types of positive emotion, which progressively neutralize or dilute the negative emotion. Through this process, the emotional pain evoked by recall of the traumatic event is slowly dissipated.

emotional pain. In this way, emotion would be progressively diluted by exposure of memories to the prevailing mood.

It has been proposed that depression and mania develop when an excess of similar emotion is transferred from the mood to memories that enter consciousness. SD has been discussed, because it seems to provide a unique opportunity to directly observe this form of emotional transfer in relative isolation. When SD is employed, nonthreatening emotion from the mood serves to dilute small amounts of negative emotion arising during directed thought. When mood disorders evolve, the same basic form of emotional transfer probably occurs, but with a different result. In these disorders, emotion is acquired in excess from prolonged moods and associates with thoughts that enter active awareness. An excess of such transferred emotion would eventually dominate any original emotion associated with such entities. As a consequence, a state of emotional polarization, rather than dilution, would result. The final outcome, of course, would depend upon the type and intensity of the transferred emotion, as well as on that already associated with cycling memories. It is therefore proposed that the principles underling SD are similar in many ways to those driving the development of mood disorders. In effect, emotion derived from the mood may produce enhancement of emotional sensitivity under some conditions and desensitization in others. Of course, the transfer of emotion down lines of association is central to both processes. The emotional changes postulated to occur in systematic desensitization are illustrated in Figure 8.6.

ANTIDEPRESSANT DRUGS

The treatment of depression with medication is also a very effective form of therapy. Antidepressant drugs are particularly effective when used in combination with psychotherapy (Weissman, 1978). These medications are thought to work by altering the transmission of neurochemicals between nerve cells. This would, of course, affect the degree to which neurons are associated with each other and suggests that antidepressants could potentially produce the same structural changes as those proposed for psychotherapy. It is worth noting that all antidepressants, regardless of chemical class, usually require several weeks before any symptomatic relief can be noted. This is consistent with a slow, gradual change, as we can imagine might occur when association patterns are changed. Perhaps this may be a part of the mechanism by which antidepressants relieve depression.

OVERVIEW

Mood disorders appear to represent a complex grouping of interrelated mental illnesses. It is therefore reasonable that any theoretical consideration of this subject would also be quiet complex. In this chapter, many separate ideas and observations concerning mood disorders have been presented. At this point, perhaps a brief overview of the key elements of this hypothesis would help further to clarify and focus these concepts.

A theory of depression and mania has been proposed. It is based upon the premise that the emotion associated with memories can change in response to life circumstances and become polarized. When a redistribution of emotional associations occurs, the fixed mood states characteristic of these disorders may be generated and maintained.

As discussed before, initial episodes of depression or mania may be precipitated by events that are perceived as emotionally stimulating. This has been observed by others (Angst, 1966; Dunner et al., 1979). This may involve a single event or perhaps many separate experiences occurring over time, which act in unison to produce a strong blend of emotion. The mood disturbance that ultimately develops, and its accompanying symptoms, seems to reflect directly the type of emotion that becomes fixated in this process. For example, mania is usually characterized by emotions that might be generally described as energizing. Such emotions as anger, euphoria, optimism, entitlement, and grandiosity are often typical of the moods observed in the illness. In contrast, emotions that are consistently dysphoric seem to produce the deenergizing and frustrating symptoms of depression. It has been proposed that the perception of fatigue experienced by most depressed patients is a direct consequence of this type of emotion. In contrast, the hyperactivity and agitated drive that characterize mania are probably a direct reflection of the nature of emotion that seems to dominate in this disorder.

In many cases, events that precipitate an episode of depression or mania may be clearly evident to an examining physician. In others, the initiating stressors may be much more obscure. As discussed before, this is often the situation in patients who have experienced prior illness. In such cases, it is presumed that some associative changes remain after each occurrence of the disorder, which may facilitate the onset of subsequent episodes. In effect, milder, less evident psychosocial stressors may produce illness if sufficient associative bias has accumulated from prior episodes. This may occur in individuals with a biological predisposition to these mood disturbances.

It is postulated that hippocampal activity is initiated in response to all emotionally stimulating events that occur. Such a response may produce memory consolidation that is proportional to the emotion experienced. Hippocampal activity would continue until the associated emotion was sufficiently diluted. As this occurred, memories of the stimulating events would progressively fade from active awareness. In other words, the issues of initial concern would gradually lose their emotional impact through dilution, allowing the brain to focus on other concerns. In some cases, such precipitating events alone or in combination with other similar experiences would generate an unusually intense degree of emotion. Under such conditions, emotional polarization, rather than dilution, might be the net result. In other words, the intensity of the original emotion would outweigh that encountered from memories utilized in subsequent thought and would become concentrated rather than dispersed. Emotion from the original stimulating events would thus be spread down lines of association to many other memories utilized in thought. The process would eventually end, but perhaps not before many associated memories had acquired some of the original emotion. Conditions favoring depression or mania would thus be generated.

When hippocampal activity is prolonged, many memories in current usage may acquire emotion from the original stimulating events. As a result, the emotion released by the frequent interpretation of such memories during routine thought would perpetuate the resulting mood state in consciousness. As explained before, the strength of such memories should also increase their frequency in thought, which would further perpetuate the existing mood. Such an arrangement would therefore favor the recall of those memories involved in the polarization process that had recently been strengthened through hippocampal activity. Under such conditions, a relatively fixed mood state characteristic of depression or one of the various types of mania might eventually be produced and maintained in consciousness.

This model predicts that polarization generally travels outward along lines of association from the original source of emotion. If the initial emotion is unusually intense, the polarization process may be widespread and involve many memories before it can be contained. With less intense emotion, some spread of original emotion probably also occurs. In such cases, dilution may be achieved more rapidly, thus greatly limiting the number of secondary memories receiving polarized emotion. The psychological technique of systematic desensitization was presented to illustrate how emotion can be acquired by memories from the mood. The progressive improvement that can be achieved with this technique is also consistent with the overall concept of emotional transfer from one memory to the next along lines of association.

Under nonpathological conditions, we can imagine that some degree of emotional polarization is probably normal. Perhaps at any given time there are numerous memories with associated emotion in various degrees of resolution. Eventually, such emotion should become dissipated through dilution, and the hippocampal cycle would slow or stop. When an emotion was very intense, it might be spread to many associated memories before being adequately contained. As indicated before, zones of polarized emotion (i.e., areas of like emotion) may be the result. Such conditions may produce the emotional lability and mixed-state characteristics of early mood disorders. If the polarization was excessive, an episode of depression or mania would eventually develop. Under rare conditions, sizable zones of opposing emotion might be generated. Relatively frequent switches from manic to depressive symptoms would be observed under these conditions, resulting in a rapid-cycling form of illness.

The relatively fixed mood states that seem to characterize depression and mania may explain many of the common symptoms of these disorders. The difficulty with memory reported by most depressed patients represents a good example. In a mental state characterized by severe mood inflexibility, memory retrieval would be greatly limited by state-dependent effects. The profound loss of insight commonly displayed by manic patients probably also represents an inability to evaluate situations adequately because of the same retrieval problems. The delusions and auditory hallucinations that are common in these syndromes may also arise from this underlying situation. Thoughts arising from memories associated with inaccessible moods might be viewed as intrusive voices, because they could not adequately be interpreted. False beliefs might be maintained because of a failure to retrieve data linked with other mood states. As indicated, mood disorders seem to arise from conditions that produce emotional inflexibility. In turn, many of the symptoms common to these disorders may result.

Miscellaneous Topics

In this chapter, an assorted group of topics will be discussed which relate, in some way, to the proposed association hypothesis and its interpretation in normal and pathological mental states.

MENTAL REPRESENTATION OF THE WORLD

Within each of us is a mental representation of the world, which is maintained and updated continuously. Generalized memories are present and serve as a system of mental classification and storage for the many events we encounter in life. When data enters the brain, it is evaluated in light of prior experience, so that it might be fully understood in terms relevant to us. As indicated, this probably involves a combination of literal and emotional interpretations. Through this process, we view things from our own unique perspective. Each event is assessed and measured in a context that has been established through repeated interpretations of past events. Each value judgment we make in this way is stored in association with the original memory and used in subsequent interpretations. Our internal representation is therefore composed of much more than a mere recording of external events. This type of cognitive processing results in a mental representation that is composed of descriptive memories of external events, combined with their interpretations. Because of variations in individual experience, each of us possesses a storehouse of knowledge that is slightly different and unique. This is why each of us may see a similar situation in a slightly different way. Each individual's view of the world is shaped by his or her internal perspective, which is a direct reflection of his or her experiences and their interpretations.

The memories that collectively form our mental representations are in a constant state of flux. New data and conclusions are constantly being added, and older material is modified or replaced. The process constantly updates itself, so that we maintain the most balanced representation possible. A simultaneous process of remembering and forgetting serves to maintain relevancy in our picture of the world. Issues of immediate importance are stored in memory and may become strengthened through repetition. If not repeated, they fade through disuse and are replaced by more current memories. In this way, the brain is able to focus on the issues at hand. Besides repetition from direct experience, the durability of memories is determined by their emotional components. Events experienced during intense emotion are frequently important and are so marked by the associated feeling. This seems to be a mechanism by which the brain ensures that significant memories will be more lasting. As postulated, the hippocampus may play a vital role in this mental function.

ATTITUDES AND VALUES

Each of us has a wide range of attitudes and values, which have evolved over time and are a part of our mental representation of the world. These entities are the product of repeated value judgments of our many experiences. We may decide to buy a certain new car, because it reminds us of previous models we have liked. This information would become available to us through the interpretation process, and would be transferred to the memory of the new car to be used in subsequent evaluations. Probably all of our likes and dislikes arise from prior experience in this way. Of course, most opinions are derived from the interpretation of several memories and therefore may be a blend of prior opinions. These mixed interpretations are probably more the rule than the exception. Through the storage of many experiences in memory, relatively stable attitudes and values may arise. They may be considered to be the product of many experiences, which have come to represent a relatively consistent point of view. Over the course of time, our preferences may change as we accumulate new experiences. The minor interpretative changes that result may cumulatively produce alterations in our attitudes and values. As indicated before, our mental representation of the world is constantly being updated to reflect our current situations in life.

For any mental representation of the world to be useful, it must faithfully reflect external events. The physical reality portrayed in our memories must be reasonably accurate for our literal interpretations to be correct. In a like manner, emotional assessments must reflect the true situation as closely as possible. Any errors generated during the interpretation process will be stored with new memories and lead to further mistakes on subsequent interpretations. Occasionally such errors probably occur but may have little overall consequence. Because most interpretations are derived from several memories in combination, a single error from one of these should cause only a slight distortion. The continual updating of information that occurs should also help to correct or dilute errors such as these. Reality testing would seem to be a critical function of the brain. Without an accurate, internal picture of the world, reality could not be appreciated, and very little meaningful activity would be possible. Psychosis probably occurs whenever there is a major imbalance between objective reality and its internal perception.

GENERALIZED KNOWLEDGE

The ideas presented here constitute a hypothesis that attempts to explain the organization of the brain based on the association of memories. In essence, the formation of associations can be viewed as a way of maintaining the natural relationships perceived through the senses. This would seem to be an important concept. The type and amount of information stored within the brain would be a direct reflection of experience. Through generalized knowledge, things would be naturally classified and maintained only as long as they had relevance to the brain. There would be nothing arbitrary or random about a system such as this. Knowledge would be added to memory stores and undergo a process of progressive consolidation into generalized knowledge. This would effectively condense information into its most usable form, as determined by experience. If a new memory continued to have current relevance as an individual entity, its conversion into generalized knowledge would be slowed. Through repetition in thought, it would become stronger because of its current usefulness. When the situation changed, and individual significance of the memory lessened, it too would slowly blend into generalized knowledge. This would be part of the ongoing process by which our internal representation of the world is updated to better reflect our situation at any given time.

LOCALIZATION OF MEMORIES

Within the brain there is a vast sea of memories that must be accessed on a regular basis. Obviously, some efficient system for the localization of single memories or GMCs must be available. Associations make this possible. They are the glue that hold smaller memories together so that larger memories can exist. Within this collection of memories, these linkages form barriers that segregate and subdivide stored information into discrete pieces of data corresponding to experience.

In this country today, there are literally millions of individual telephones. Each can by accessed by an area code combined with a seven-digit number. In essence, each has a single 10-digit number that specifically sets it apart from all others. In a sense, memories may be analogous to telephone numbers. Each of the 10 digits might be thought of as a GMC composing a larger memory. Each such memory would be held together by the association of its individual pieces, Incoming data would be broken down into their smallest component parts, which would correspond to GMCs. In combination, these would specify a given larger memory in the same way a 10-digit phone number designates a single telephone out of millions. Of course, memories contain no set number of component GMCs. If two GMCs are unique to a given larger memory, they may be sufficient to trigger the whole entity. In other cases, many GMCs might be necessary to designate a memory, because their combination may be common to many memories. This system works only because of the association that links memories together. Larger memories can only be localized because they contain certain discrete parts, specified by their simultaneous grouping in nature and held together by association linkages.

To complete a long distance call, a three-digit area code must first be dialed. These codes group individual telephone numbers into clusters to facilitate their access. In the above analogy, this three-digit code might be thought of as the emotion associated with memories. To locate a given memory, its emotional code must first be correctly matched before the remainder of the memory can be identified. Like area codes, emotional associations may serve to organize memories into groups to facilitate the localization process.

LITERAL AND EMOTIONAL INTERPRETATIONS

It is probable that everything that enters our senses is evaluated at some level. In many cases, this may occur out of active awareness. Many things that are routine and require no immediate action may never reach consciousness. These probably represent literal identifications of situations and objects we encounter on a regular basis. Little or no emotional component may be present. The absence of emotion may signify events of lesser significance and prevent their entry into active consciousness.

Other interpretations may be both literal and emotional. This would provide physical recognition, as well as any emotional importance determined from prior experience. These are the types of interpretations that seem most likely to enter consciousness. This system probably protects the conscious brain from an overwhelming volume of trivial information, enabling it to deal with issues of more significance. A mechanism by which conscious and unconscious mental activity might coexist is presented in the following paragraphs.

SPONTANEOUS DEPOLARIZATION OF NEURONS

Most cells in the central nervous system exhibit a continuous, slow rate of spontaneous depolarization. This effect can be demonstrated with tiny electrodes, thinner than an average nerve-cell body (Eccles, 1964). Insertion of such microelectrodes into cells in various areas of the cortex indicates that the spontaneous rate of decay varies from one region to the next. Frequencies ranging from about 1 impulse per second to a 100 or more have been recorded. Cumulatively, these impulses compose the electrical activity recorded with an electroencephalogram. This form of periodic discharge seems to be an intrinsic characteristic of most nerve cells. This fascinating subject is discussed by Llinas in his 1990 article.

Spontaneous depolarization does not appear to be dependent upon outside influences. It can be observed in isolated nerve tissue as readily as cells in vivo. In cells receiving a sensory input, a change in this natural rate of oscillation can often be observed. This effect is generally thought to reflect the information present in the input. In other words, a change in rate may convey some meaning to the brain about the original sensory input. For example, physical movement can be sensed by the vestibular apparatus in the inner ear and translated into variations in nerve impulse. If an electrode is inserted into the vestibular nerve of the monkey, the spontaneous rate of depolarization will increase if the monkey is turned in one direction and decrease if rotation is in the other direction. Thus, bodily movement, which is sensed physically within the fluid-filled channels of the inner ear, is translated into changes in discharge rate of this cranial nerve, providing the brain with information on movement (Hudspeth & Corey, 1977). It is now generally accepted that most sensory input, such as the loudness of a sound or brightness of a light, is encoded by changes in the basic rate of oscillation of sensory cells.

DEPOLARIZATION OF LOCALIZED MEMORY STRUCTURES

Perhaps memories, as electrically coherent, neural units, also have intrinsic rates of spontaneous discharge that can change upon activation. In the localization process, many separate inputs may be received almost simultaneously by a memory, producing its activation as an intact whole. We can speculate that this may produce an overall increase in the baseline level of depolarization for such structures. In other words, when a memory is activated during the localization process, its depolarization rate may change to reflect the input. It is reasonable to assume that this may be a graded response. In other words, memories containing only a few component GMCs or subunits may experience only partial activation, whereas those that are more completely matched may be much more vigorously stimulated. If these assumptions are basically correct, then several aspects of mental activity might be explained, as will be discussed.

In the localization process proposed here, many structures other than those composing the identified memory would receive some energy and achieve some degree of activation. This would be an unavoidable consequence of the process as described. Incoming sensory information would trigger matching structures, which, in turn, would produce activation of their associations, and so forth. Energy would be spread in exponential fashion through many levels of neurons. This widely divergent wave of activation would ultimately touch many memories. Many larger entities, containing only a few component structures, would be partially activated, whereas others might be more completely matched and more highly activated. Presumably the structures with the most matching components would be the most highly stimulated and would preferentially enter consciousness.

It is obvious that a system such as this would produce a great deal of neural depolarization, which would occur almost simultaneously during localization. Some way would be needed to distinguish the most strongly activated entities from the background noise produced by memories with lesser degrees of stimulation. This could perhaps be accomplished if we assume that the rate of impulse discharge following activation is directly related to the degree of stimulation received by the structure. In other words, the most completely matched entity would be the most highly activated, and would experience the greatest rate of electrical depolarization. All activated structures would show an increased rate of discharge, but the ones with the highest degree of stimulation would experience the most vigorous rate of reverberation. In some way, this might designate the memory structures most closely corresponding to incoming data.

THRESHOLD FREQUENCY AND CONSCIOUSNESS

Perhaps there is a threshold frequency for depolarization that must be exceeded for a memory to enter consciousness. This might be one of several possible ways that the background noise of mental activity could be prevented from entering awareness, while still allowing the most highly activated memories to be sensed. In effect, some form of neural filtration system may allow only those memories with the highest levels of activation to gain access to consciousness. In this way, a large number of memories that may experience only partial activation in the localization process would be excluded from consciousness.

It also seems reasonable to assume that much of the background noise generated during the localization process may be attenuated to some extent by lateral inhibition. Even though this phenomenon has been extensively investigated in the visual system, inhibitory circuits that perform this same basic function have been identified in many other areas of the brain. Indeed, at least half of the synaptic connections that have been studied appear to be inhibitory in nature. Lateral inhibition, which is known as surround inhibition or center-surround antagonism in visual pathways, refers to the ability of a cell with a large output to inhibit its neighbors with lower outputs. The net result of this effect appears to be an exaggeration of the natural differences between cell outputs, allowing a single strong signal to be effectively focused. Perhaps memories, as clusters of electrically interwoven neurons, are also capable of some form of lateral inhibition. In other words, full activation of such structures may inhibit other memories that are less strongly stimulated, as is postulated to occur during the localization process. In 1989, Calvin suggested that such an effect may help in the selection of data arising from several tracks of information being simultaneously processed at an unconscious level. Through this mechanism, lateral inhibition may facilitate the selection and entry of strongly activated memories into consciousness. These ideas suggest that if a frequency threshold exists, it may represent a balance between the signal strengths of memories that receive stimulation during thought or sensory perception and the ability of lateral inhibition to dissipate background noise, so that a single entity may emerge in consciousness.

LATERAL INHIBITION AS A BASIS FOR CONCENTRATION

If lateral inhibition is a general property of memories, it may provide a basis for our ability to concentrate. Consider the following theoretical argument in support of this idea: When we try to recall something that is not immediately available in consciousness, our mental focus seems to narrow in an attempt to isolate the subject in question. For example, we may try to recall the name of an actor who recently appeared in a movie or television program. His mental image, as well as other known details about this individual, may be recalled and cycled through consciousness repeatedly in an effort to remember the associated name. This process may continue for several minutes or longer and seems to be a general technique utilized by people when they intentionally try to remember. As a consequence of this process, other thoughts and memories, not immediately related to this subject, seem to be excluded from consciousness. This, of course, probably facilitates the recall of the desired memories by reducing background noise. It seems possible that the memories we consider in this process may be strongly stimulated, and the lateral inhibition that results may minimize the activation and recall of unrelated memories. In effect, background distraction would be reduced, allowing the brain to focus more clearly on the issues at hand. Under these conditions, the memory of the name, which is associated with the other memories of this individual, may be more readily activated and called into consciousness. Through this process, lateral inhibition may produce what we generally regard as concentration.

OTHER THEORIES OF NEURAL OSCILLATION

Other theories have also suggested that the rhythmic, electrical activity inherent to nerve cells may, in some way, mediate conscious awareness. In 1990, Crick and Koch proposed that changes in the natural pattern of neural oscillation may allow visual images to gain entrance into consciousness. These authors envisioned the cerebral cortex as composed of cells that randomly oscillate at a baseline frequency of about 40 Hz. In response to a visual perception, the random oscillation arising from its neural components becomes synchronized or phase-locked. Information depicted in the image is conveyed to consciousness without an increase in the rate of cellular oscillation. Such an arrangement circumvents the theoretical problem of image superposition, which may exist in some visual systems. Through the process of synchronization, the individual cell assemblies composing the image undergo binding and acquire sufficient coherence to enter conscious awareness.

CONSCIOUS AND UNCONSCIOUS NEURAL ACTIVITY

In the work presented here, a system of mental organization based on the association of memories has been postulated. It relies heavily on the concept that we only understand things because of prior experience. Everything is evaluated in light of memories stored largely as generalized knowledge. Both literal and emotional interpretations are mixed to provide understanding of new data. Much of this mental activity is postulated to occur out of our awareness. In the system presented here, consciousness has been described as a cyclic flow of ideas passing through the unconscious interpretative areas into the sensory perception areas. Through this route, the results of the unconscious information processing may enter conscious awareness. This combination of unconscious and conscious information manipulation may function together to produce the mental activity we utilize as humans. The proposals presented in the previous paragraphs may help to understand how this might be possible.

The idea that many forms of mental activity occur out of the reach of conscious awareness is certainly not new. This concept is usually attributed to Sigmund Freud. The hypothesis proposed here is generally in agreement with this speculation. As indicated earlier, there do appear to be mental processes that occur without our conscious knowledge. The composition of sentences, the translation of language into tangible images, and the interpretation of new data all seem to represent examples of this type of activity. The concept of a frequency threshold isolating some mental activity from consciousness might provide an explanation for this effect. Perhaps the memories and neural circuits that accomplish unconscious functions operate at subthreshold frequencies, thus shielding the bulk of this activity from consciousness. As proposed before, normal thought seems to combine both conscious and unconscious processes in a cyclic manner. This system may allow routine work to be accomplished without interfering with the higher functions conducted in consciousness. Conscious and unconscious mental activity may be possible if such a frequency threshold exists.

SHORT-TERM MEMORY

As proposed in this hypothesis, when new data are taken into the brain, or when thought is circulated, a localization and matching process occurs, in which the most similar memory or combination of memories is identified. This process may serve as the initiation for short-term memory. When structures localized in this way become activated, their spontaneous rate of depolarization may increase, as suggested in the preceding paragraphs. This oscillating impulse may constitute our perception of the events in question, and may remain in consciousness as long as the depolarization rate remained above the threshold frequency. Conscious awareness of the thought or memory would fade when the oscillating impulse decayed below this frequency. This decay process might require only seconds to a minute or so but should provide us with ample time for consideration of the entity in most routine cases. The perception of this decaying impulse may be what we recognize as short-term memory.

After the repetitive impulse of short-term memory dropped below the threshold frequency, decay might continue for some time. The memory would no longer be present in consciousness but might still be oscillating at a rate greater than its intrinsic resting frequency. As long as some excess depolarization occurred, the memory might be more easily triggered back into consciousness than in the resting state. This may explain the phenomenon of repetitive priming, described earlier. This term refers to the observation that recently presented material seems to be more easily recalled than nonpresented material when subtle cues are given as retrieval stimuli. We can speculate that when newly presented data leave consciousness, this data may still oscillate for some time at a frequency above that of the resting memory. Under these conditions, a subtle cue might provide enough energy to increase the depolarization rate above the frequency threshold, producing reentry of the memory into consciousness. Nonpresented data would be at rest and have a lower oscillation rate. More energy would therefore be required to boost it past the consciousness barrier. Such a memory would therefore be more difficult to retrieve when a limited amount of input data was available. The concept of a frequency threshold separating conscious from unconscious processes is illustrated in Figure 9.1.

Without the temporal limitations of short-term memory, thoughts and evoked memories might accumulate in consciousness for long periods of time. Normal cognitive processes might be greatly impaired by the confusion and chaos that would seem inherent in such a system. This suggests a rationale for limiting the duration of memories in consciousness. In contrast, emotions seem capable of blending to produce a single emotional tone or mood. Unlike memories, they appear to be sensed cumulatively and can coexist with normal thought without producing confusion. In fact, the simultaneous presence of thought and emotion in consciousness may be necessary for full interpretation, as discussed. Cu-

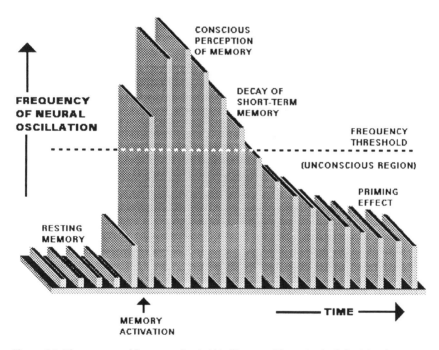

Figure 9.1 The concept of *frequency threshold* is illustrated here. At the left of this figure, the oscillation of resting memories at a low intrinsic rate is shown. At the point of memory activation, this frequency increases until it exceeds the threshold for consciousness. For a short period of time, a spontaneous decay in this frequency occurs above the threshold, which correlates with short-term memory. Below the threshold, the memory is no longer in active consciousness. In this region, the rate of frequency decay slows but eventually returns to the resting baseline. These residual reverberations of this memory below the threshold may facilitate the priming effect, as discussed in the text.

mulative emotion, sensed as the mood, seems to provide a current emotional reference that frames and influences our thoughts and their interpretations. If emotions were subject to the same short-term limitations as memories, this form of contextual reference might not be available to reflect the current emotional status.

THE HIPPOCAMPUS AND NEURAL OSCILLATION RATE

It was suggested earlier that the hippocampus may function to repetitively activate memories that are associated with emotion. This may serve to consolidate new memories and to strengthen older ones that acquire new emotion. This effect may work in tandem with the increase in oscillation rate, which has been postulated to occur when a memory is initially localized and activated. If emotion is released during this process, the hippocampus may perpetuate the resulting increase in depolarization rate. As a consequence, the retention of an emotional memory in consciousness may be enhanced somewhat. This may explain the general observation that emotional thoughts seem to remain in consciousness longer than those that are more routine and less emotionally charged.

It seems possible that hippocampal activity may also drive the consolidation of emotionally charged memories after they leave active consciousness. When emotionally stimulating events occur, memories and thoughts may be generated that can dominate consciousness for relatively long periods of time. As such entities begin to experience emotional dilution, their rate of oscillation may diminish somewhat, allowing them to pass out of consciousness. In the unconsciousness realm, it is conceivable that hippocampal-mediated consolidation may continue. Even though such entities may no longer be visible in active consciousness, they should still be more easily retrievable than other memories in storage because of the priming effect produced by ongoing hippocampal activity. In such a state, fewer cues would be required for their activation, which would serve to keep them close to consciousness.

EMOTION FROM UNCONSCIOUS
INFORMATION PROCESSING

Although memories experiencing unconscious activation via hippocampal activity may remain out of consciousness, the emotion released during this process may still be capable of influencing the mood. This is based on the assumption that emotions, unlike memories, seem to be experienced in an additive manner. It is conceivable that small amounts of similar emotion, released over time through continual hippocampal activity, may cumulatively achieve the strength necessary to enter consciousness, even though their parent memories may remain unconscious. This may explain why subjective mismatches between conscious thought and displays of emotion can occasionally be observed. For example, mildly depressed patients often report spontaneous crying for reasons they cannot explain, and individuals with anxiety disorders may experience seemingly unprovoked panic attacks. Many examples in which unconscious mental activity appears to exert some influence on conscious thought can be cited. Perhaps such effects are produced when memories are activated unconsciously, and cumulative emotion finds its way into consciousness, as described here.

Earlier, it was noted that emotion seems to be capable of lingering in the background for long periods of time after the associated memory has passed from consciousness. The cumulative perception of this quality seems to constitute our mood. Perhaps this can be explained by assuming that at least part of the emotion that constitutes an existing mood originates from the unconscious processing of memories that continue to oscillate below the consciousness threshold, as discussed earlier. In other words, a memory may fade from consciousness, but its continued unconscious processing may still contribute emotion to the mood. Emotion may therefore only appear to linger in consciousness after the parent memory has passed from active awareness. In reality, such emotion may actually be generated and released continuously into the mood by unconscious activity, producing the illusion that it lingers after a memory has faded from consciousness.

SWITCHING AS A GENERAL PHENOMENON

From the ideas presented in this work, a theoretical bridge linking mood disorders and multiple personality disorder (MPD) can be established. The most basic assumption to this proposal is that MPD and affective disorders both arise from isolated clusters of memories tightly associated with a narrow grouping of emotions. As a consequence of this arrangement, emotions may be expressed that produce and maintain the pathological moods observed in these disorders.

Under such conditions, abrupt changes in mood content may occur, allowing access to new sets of memories. In MPD, such switching may result in the appearance of alternate personality structures. In affective disorders, functionally analogous transitions in the dominant emotional state may result in mood swings. It is even conceivable that complete transitions from depression to mania and vice versa may represent a form of this phenomenon. These observations suggest that switching may be a general psychological process, arising, at least in part, from the isolated conditions postulated to exist in both conditions.

In his 1989 book entitled Multiple Personality: Diagnosis, Clinical Features, and Treatment, Colin Ross takes a similar position. He suggests that unipolar depression represents a dissociation of the normal mood state, and that recovery occurs through a switching process similar to that occurring in MPD. Depression and the normal euthymic state are thus viewed as analogous to alter personalities. He also suggests, "Manic–depressive illness is a disorder of switching. Patients with the disorder switch states in a pathological manner. Their problem is severalfold: They switch into states, switch out of states, and get stuck in states in an abnormal manner" (p. 173). These ideas are consistent with the concept that depression and mania may originate from relatively isolated pockets of memories, which may actually coexist with each other under certain conditions. This, of course, may be particularly useful in understanding the phenomenon of rapid and ultrarapid cycling. Although Ross's ideas and those presented here originate from different theoretical considerations, both seem to point in the same general direction.

In further support of these ideas, Ross indicates that clinical depression in MPD patients may be restricted to one or two alters, while other personalities structures may remain euthymic. This strongly suggests that depression is not the result of some global influence on mental function. In contrast, it seems more likely that depression arises through discrete changes in neural architecture, involving a relatively small number of memories. This, of course, is consistent with the proposal that mood disorders may arise when groupings of memories acquire a single blending of associated emotion. As a result of this process, relatively isolated pockets of memories may be generated, from which the pathology of MPD and mood disorders may originate.

Ross views dissociation as a general mental process that is not solely restricted to pathological processes such as MPD and mood disorders. He suggests that this phenomenon may be a common and frequent part of normal mental function, which occurs during daydreaming and numerous other forms of cognitive activity requiring concentration. The theoretical construct presented here suggests that this is a reasonable assumption. It is proposed that dissociation, in its simplest form, occurs every time there is a change in mood composition. In normal individuals, such switching would occur frequently and easily in response to incoming information or internal stimuli. In most cases, such transitions in mood would be gradual and fluid. As a consequence, access to the different memories, necessary for the support of normal cognitive function, would be perceived as smooth and continuous. In pathological conditions, the degree to which emotion is shared between memories may be reduced; that is, domains of memories associated with polarized emotion may have evolved as described in earlier chapters. As a result, mood flexibility may be reduced, and switching might be more pronounced and discontinuous. Access to memories other than those associated with the existing mood may be much more restricted. Under such conditions, there would actually be a reduction in cognitive perspective, as compared with the normal state. In some cases, a significant degree of amnesia for memories associated with other mood states may occur, producing symptoms of psychosis, as explained before. It is therefore suggested that changes in mood composition that occur under non-pathological conditions represent a form of dissociation that is necessary for normal cognitive function. When conditions of emotional segregation evolve during mental illness, this normal process may become more obvious and appear pathological.

CONCLUDING REMARKS

Much speculation is obviously inherent to any hypothesis such as this. Even so, the ideas presented seem rational and have an internal consistency, which suggest some degree of plausibility. Of course, both time and research will be necessary to fully evaluate the concepts presented. Perhaps the general principles of this hypothesis would be amenable to computer modeling. This is a fascinating idea, because it might provide a more tangible way to evaluate the relationships postulated. This approach, in combination with conventional laboratory and clinical research, should eventually allow many of the ideas in this work to be tested. It is hoped that this hypothesis will eventually lead to a better understanding of the human brain. Only through this type of knowledge can mental illness be fully comprehended and a more rational basis for treatment be established.

References

Abrams, R., & Taylor, M.A. (1981). Importance of schizophrenic symptoms in the diagnosis of mania. *American Journal of Psychiatry, 138,* 658–661.

Ackley, D.H., Hinton, G.E., & Sejnowski, T.J. (1985). A learning algorithm for Boltzmann machines. *Cognitive Science, 9,* 147–169.

Akiskal, H.S. (1983). The bipolar spectrum: New concepts in classification and diagnosis. In L. Grinspoon (Ed.), *Psychiatry update* (Vol. 2, pp. 271–292). Washington, DC: American Psychiatric Press.

Akiskal, H.S., Yerevanian, B.I., Davis, G.C., King, D., & Lemmi, H. (1985). The nosologic status of borderline personality: Clinical and polysomnographic study. *American Journal of Psychiatry, 142,* 192–198.

Allman, W.F. (1989). *Apprentices of wonder: Inside the neural network revolution.* New York: Bantam Books.

American Psychiatric Association. (1987). *Diagnostic and statistical manual of mental disorders* (3rd Ed. Rev.). Washington, DC: Author.

Anderson, J.A. (1970). Two models for memory organization using interacting traces. *Mathematical Biosciences, 8,* 137–160.

Anderson, J.R., & Bower, G.H. (1972). *Human associative memory.* Washington, DC: Winston.

Andorfer, J.C. (1985). Multiple personality in the human information-processor: A case history and theoretical formulation. *Journal of Clinical Psychology, 41,* 309–324.

Andreasen, N.C. (1984). *The broken brain.* New York: Harper & Row.

Angst, J. (1966). *Zur Atiologie und Nosologie endogener depressiver Psychosen.* Berlin: Springer.

Angst, J., Weis, P., Grof, P., Baastrup, P.C., & Schou, M. (1970). Lithium prophylaxis in recurrent affective disorders. *British Journal of Psychiatry, 116,* 604–614.

Angyal, A. (1941). *Foundations for a science of personality.* Cambridge, MA: Harvard University Press.

Antrobus, J.S., Singer, J.L., Goldstein, S., & Fortgang, M. (1970). Mindwandering and cognitive structure. *Transactions of the New York Academy of Sciences, 32,* 242–252.

Baastrup, P.C., & Schou, M. (1967). Lithium as a prophylactic agent. *Archives of General Psychiatry, 16,* 162–172.

Baddeley, A. (1986). *Working memory.* Oxford: Clarendon Press.

Bard, P. (1938). Studies in the cortical representation of somatic sensibility. *Harvey Lectures, 33,* 143–169.

Barnes, C.A. (1979). Memory deficits associated with senescence: A neurophysiological and behavioral study of the rat. *Journal of Comparative and Physiological Psychology, 93,* 74–104.

Bass, M.J., & Hull, C.L. (1934). Irradiation of a tactile conditioned reflex in man. *Journal of Comparative and Physiological Psychology, 17,* 47–65.

Bauer, R.M. (1986). The cognitive psychophysiology of prosopagnosia. In H. Ellis, M. Jeeves, F. Newcombe, & A. Young (Eds.). *Aspects of face processing* (pp. 253–267). Dordrecht, The Netherlands: Martinus Nijhoff.

Baxter, L.R., Jr., Phelps, M.E., Mazziotta, J.C., Schwartz, J.M., Gerner, R.H., Selin, C.E., & Sumida, R.M. (1985). Cerebral metabolic rates for glucose in mood disorders: Studies with positron emission tomography and fluorodeoxyglucose F 18. *Archives of General Psychiatry, 42,* 441–447.

Beck, A.T., Rush, A.J., Shaw, B.F., & Emery, G. (1979). *Cognitive therapy of depression.* New York, Guilford.

Beigel, A., & Murphy, D.L. (1971). Assessing clinical characteristics of the manic state. *American Journal of Psychiatry, 128,* 688–694.

Bennett, E.L., Krech, D., & Rosenzweig, M.R. (1964). Reliability and regional specificity of cerebral effects of environmental complexity and training. *Journal of Comparative and Physiological Psychology, 57,* 440–441.

Berger, W.F., & Thompson, R.F. (1978a). Neuronal plasticity in the limbic system during classical conditioning of the rabbit nictitating membrane response: I. Hippocampus. *Brain Research, 145,* 323–346.

Berger, W.F., & Thompson, R.F. (1978b). Neuronal plasticity in the limbic system during classical conditioning of the rabbit nictitating membrane response: II. Septum and mammillary bodies. *Brain Research, 156,* 293–314.

Black, D.W., & Nasrallah, A. (1989). Hallucinations and delusions in 1,715 patients with unipolar and bipolar affective disorders. *Psychopathology, 22,* 28–34.

Black, D.W., Winokur, G., & Nasrallah, A. (1987). Treatment of mania: A naturalistic study of electroconvulsive therapy versus lithium in 438 patients. *Journal of Clinical Psychiatry, 48,* 132–139.

Bliss, E.L. (1980). Multiple personalities: Report of fourteen cases with implications for schizophrenia and hysteria. *Archives of General Psychiatry, 37,* 1388–1397.

Bliss, E.L. (1984). A symptom profile of patients with multiple personalities, including MMPI results. *Journal of Nervous and Mental Disease, 172,* 197–202.

Bliss, E.L. (1986). *Multiple personality, allied disorders, and hypnosis.* New York: Oxford University Press.

Bliss, E.L., Larson, E.M., & Nakashima, S.R. (1983). Auditory hallucinations and schizophrenia. *Journal of Nervous and Mental Disease, 171,* 30–33.

Bliss, T.V.P., & Garner–Medwin, R. (1973). Long-lasting potentiation of synaptic transmission in the dentate area of the unanaesthetized rabbit following stimulation of the perforant path. *Journal of Physiology, 232,* 357–374.

Bliss, T.V.P., & Lomo, T. (1973). Long-lasting potentiation of synaptic transmission in the dentate area of the unanaesthetized rabbit following stimulation of the perforant path. *Journal of Physiology, 232,* 331–356.

Bower, G.H. (1981). Mood and memory. *American Psychologist, 36,* 129–148.

Bower, G.H., Gilligan, S.G., & Monteiro, K.P. (1981). Selectivity of learning caused by affective states. *Journal of Experimental Psychology: General, 110,* 451–473.

Bower, G.H., & Hilgard, E.R. (1981). *Theories of learning* (5th ed.). Englewood Cliffs, NJ: Prentice-Hall.

Bower, G.H., Monteiro, K.P., & Gilligan, S.G. (1978). Emotional mood as a context for learning and recall. *Journal of Verbal Learning and Verbal Behavior, 17,* 573–585.

Braun, B.G. (1984). Towards a theory of multiple personality and other dissociative phenomena. *Psychiatric Clinics of North America, 7,* 171–193.

Brende, J.O. (1984). The psychophysiologic manifestations of dissociation. *Psychiatric Clinics of North America, 7,* 41–50.

Burke, M., & Mathews, A. (1992). Autobiographical memory and clinical anxiety. *Cognition and Emotion, 6,* 23–36.

Cahill, L., & McGaugh, J.L. (1990). Amygdaloid complex lesions differentially affect retention of tasks using appetitive and aversive reinforcement. *Behavioral Neuroscience, 104,* 523–543.

Calvin, W.H. (1989). *The cerebral symphony: Seashore reflections on the structure of consciousness.* New York: Bantam Books.

Cannon, W.B. (1929). *Bodily changes in pain, hunger, fear and rage.* New York: Appleton-Century-Crofts.

Carlson, G., & Strober, M. (1979). Affective disorders in adolescence. *Psychiatric Clinics of North America, 2,* 511–526.

Castellucci, V., & Kandel, E.R. (1976). Presynaptic sensitization as a mechanism for behavioral sensitization in Aplysia. *Science, 194,* 1176–1178.

Changeux, J.-P. (1985). *Neuronal man: The biology of the mind.* New York: Oxford University Press.

Churchland, P.M. (1988). *Matter and consciousness: A contemporary introduction to the philosophy of mind* (Rev. Ed.). Cambridge, MA: Bradford Books/MIT Press.

Churchland, P.S., & Sejnowski, T.J. (1992). *The computational brain.* Cambridge, MA: Bradford Books/MIT Press.

Clark, D.M., & Teasdale, J.D. (1981). Diurnal variation in clinical depression and accessibility of positive and negative experiences. *Journal of Abnormal Psychology, 91,* 87–95.

Clower, R.P., Zola-Morgan, S., & Squire, L.R. (1990). Lesions of the perirhinal cortex, but not lesions of the amygdala, exacerbate memory impairment in monkeys following lesions of the hippocampal formation. *Society for Neuroscience Abstracts, 16,* 616.

Coons, P.M., & Sterne, A.L. (1986). Initial and follow-up psychological testing on a group of patients with multiple personality disorder. *Psychological Reports, 58,* 43–49.

Cooper, L.N. (1974). A possible organization of animal memory and learning. In B. Lundquist and S. Lundquist (Eds.), *Proceedings of the Nobel Symposium on Collective Properties of Physical Systems* (pp. 252–264). New York: Academic Press.

Corballis, M.C. (1989). Laterality and human evolution. *Psychological Review, 96,* 492–505.

Crick, F., & Koch, C. (1990). Some reflections on visual awareness. In E. Kandel, T. Sejnowski, C. Stevens, & J. Watson (Eds.). *Cold Spring Harbor Symposia on Quantitative Biology: The Brain* (Vol. 55, pp. 953–962). New York: ColdSpring Harbor Press.

Crick, F., & Koch, C. (1992, September). The problem of consciousness. *Scientific American Magazine,* 152–159.

Damasio, A. (1990). Category-related recognition defects as a clue to the neural substrates of knowledge. *Trends in Neurosciences, 13,* 95–98.

Damasio, A., & Damasio, H. (1992, September). Brain and language. *Scientific American Magazine,* 88–95.

Damasio, A., Damasio, H., Tranel, D., & Brandt, J. (1990). The neural regionalization of knowledge access. In E. Kandel, T. Sejnowski, C. Stevens, & J. Watson (Eds.). *Cold Spring Harbor Symposium on Quantitative Biology: The Brain* (Vol. 55, pp. 1039–1047). New York: ColdSpring Harbor Press.

Damasio, A., Tranel, D., & Damasio, H. (1990b). Face agnosia and the neural substrates of memory. *Annual Review of Neuroscience, 13,* 89–110.

Darwin, C.R. (1965). *The expression of emotion in man and animals.* Chicago: University of Chicago Press. (Original published in 1872.)

Davidson, R.J., & Schwartz, G.E. (1977). Brain mechanisms subserving self-generated imagery: Electrophysiological specificity and patterning. *Psychophysiology, 14*, 598–601.

Davis, H. (1979a). Self-reference and the encoding of personal information in depression. *Cognitive Therapy Research, 3*, 97–110.

Davis, H., (1979b). The self-schema and subjective organization of personal information in depression. *Cognitive Therapy Research, 3*, 415–425.

Davis, M. (1992). The role of the amygdala in conditioned fear. In J. Aggleton, (Ed.), *The amygdala: Neurobiological aspects of emotion, memory, and mental dysfunction* (pp. 255–305). New York: Wiley-Liss.

Delgado, J.M.R., Roberts, W.W., & Miller, M.E. (1954). Learning motivated by electrical stimulation of the brain. *American Jouranl of Physiology, 179*, 587–593.

DeRivera, J.A. (1977). *A structural theory of the emotions.* New York: International Universities Press.

Desmond, N.L., & Levy, W.B. (1983). Synaptic correlates of associative potentiation/depression: An ultrastructural study in the hippocampus. *Brain Research, 265*, 21–30.

Diamond, D.M., Dunwiddie, T.V., & Ross, G.M. (1988). Characteristics of hippocampal primed burst potentiation *in-vitro* and in the awake rat. *Journal of Neuroscience, 8*, 4079–4088.

Duncan, C.P. (1949). The retroactive effect of electroshock on learning. *Journal of Comparative and Physiological Psychology, 42*, 32–44.

Dunner, D.L., Murphy, D., Stallone, F., & Fieve, R.R. (1979). Episode frequency prior to lithium treatment in bipolar manic–depressive patients. *Comprehensive Psychiatry, 20*, 511–515.

Dysken, M.W. (1979). Clinical usefulness of sodium amobarbital interviewing. *Archives of General Psychiatry, 36*, 789–794.

Eccles, J.C. (1964). *The physiology of synapses.* Berlin: Springer.

Edelman, G.M. (1989). *The remembered present: A biological theory of consciousness.* New York: Basic Books.

Eibl-Eibesfeldt, I. (1970). *Ethology: The Biology of behavior* (E. Klinghammer, trans.). New York: Holt, Rinehart & Winston.

Eichenbaum, H., Otto, T., & Cohen, N.J. (1991). The hippocampus—What does it do? *Behavioral and Neural Biology, 57*, 2–36.

Etcoff, N.L., Freeman, R., & Cave, K.R. (1991). Can we lose memories of faces? Content specificity and awareness in a prosopagnosic. *Journal of Cognitive Neuroscience, 3*, 25–41.

Farah, M. (1984). The neurological basis of mental imagery: A componential analysis. *Cognition, 18*, 245–272.

Farthing, G.W. (1992). *The psychology of consciousness.* Englewood Cliffs, NJ: Prentice-Hall.

Fawcett, J. (1993). Building bridges across domains of knowledge (Editorial). *Psychiatric Annals, 23* (10), 541–542.

Fogarty, S.J., & Hemsley, D.R. (1983). Depression and accessibility of memories: A longitudinal study. *British Journal of Psychiatry, 142*, 232–237.

Frijda, N.H. (1986). *The emotions.* Cambridge, UK: Cambridge University Press.

Fukushima, K. (1980). Neocognitron: A self-organizing neural network model for a mechanism of pattern recognition unaffected by shift in position. *Biological Cybernetics, 36*, 193–202.

Georgotas, A., & Cancro, R. (eds.). (1988). *Depression and mania.* New York: Elsevier.

Gershon, E.S., & Rieder, R.O. (1992, September). Major disorders of mind and brain. *Scientific American Magazine*, 126–133.

Globus, A., Rosenzweig, M.R., Bennett, E.L., & Diamond, M.C. (1973). Effects of differential experience on dendritic spine counts in rat cerebral cortex. *Journal of Comparative and Physiological Psychology, 82,* 175–181.

Godden, D.R., & Baddeley, A.D. (1975). Context-dependent memory in two natural environments: On land and underwater. *British Journal of Psychology, 66,* 325–331.

Goldenberg, G., Steiner, M., Podreka, I., & Deeke, L. (1992). Regional cerebral blood flow patterns related to verification of low- and high-imagery sentences. *Neuropsychologia, 30,* 581–586.

Goldman-Rakic, P.S. (1992, September). Working memory and the mind. *Scientific American Magazine,* 110–117.

Goodwin, D.W., Powell, B., Bremer, D., Hoine, H., & Stern, J. (1969). Alcohol and recall: State-dependent effects in man. *Science, 163,* 1358–1360.

Goodwin, F.K., & Jamison, K.R. (1990). *Manic–depressive illness.* New York: Oxford University Press.

Graf, P., & Schacter, D.L. (1985). Implicit and explicit memory for new associations in normal and amnesic subjects. *Journal of Experimental Psychology: Learning, Memory, and Cognition, 11,* 501–518.

Gray, T.S. (1989). Autonomic neuropeptide connections of the amygdala. In Y. Tache, J.E. Morley, & M.R. Brown (Eds.), *Neuropeptides and stress* (Vol. 1, pp. 92–106). New York: Springer-Verlag.

Gregory, R.L. (Ed.). (1987). *The Oxford companion to the mind.* New York: Oxford University Press.

Gunderson, J.G., & Elliott, G.R. (1985). The interface between borderline personality disorder and affective disorder. *American Journal of Psychiatry, 142,* 277–288.

Guthrie, E.R. (1935). *The psychology of learning.* New York: Harper & Row.

Hall, R.C.W., LeCann, A.F., & Schoolar, J.C. (1978). Amobarbital treatment of multiple personality. *Journal of Nervous and Mental Disease, 166,* 666–670.

Hasher, L., Rose, K.C., Zacks, R.T., Sanft, H., & Doren, B. (1985). Mood, recall and selectivity effects in college students. *Journal of Experimental Psychology: General, 114,* 104–118.

Hebb, D.O. (1949). *The organization of behavior.* New York: Wiley.

Henry, G.M., Weingartner, H., & Murphy, D.L. (1971). Idiosyncratic patterns of learning and word association during mania. *American Journal of Psychiatry, 128,* 564–574.

Hilgard, E.R., & Bower, G.H. (1975). *Theories of learning* (4th ed.). Englewood Cliffs, NJ: Prentice-Hall.

Himmelhoch, J.M., Mulla, D., Neil, J.F., Detre, T.P., & Kupfer, D.J. (1976). Incidence and significance of mixed affective states in a bipolar population. *Archives of General Psychiatry, 33,* 1062–1066.

Hinton, G.E. (1992, September). How neural networks learn from experience. *Scientific American Magazine,* 144–151.

Hintzman, D.L. (1992). Mathematical constraints on the Tulving–Wiseman law. *Psychological Review, 102,* 536–542.

Hitchcock, J.M., & Davis, M. (1987). Fear-potentiated startle using an auditory conditioned stimulus: Effect of lesions of the amygdala. *Physiology and Behavior, 39,* 403–408.

Ho, B.T., Richards, D.W., & Chute, D.L. (1978). *Drug discrimination and state dependent learning.* New York: Academic Press.

Hopfield, J.J. (1982). Neural networks and physical systems with emergent collective computational abilities. *Proceedings of the National Academy of Sciences USA, 79,* 2554–2558.

Horel, J.A. (1978). The neuroanatomy of amnesia: A critique of the hippocampal memory hypothesis. *Brain, 101,* 403–445.

Hovland, C.I. (1937). The generalization of conditioned responses: I. The sensory generalization of conditioned responses with varying frequencies of tone. *Journal of General Psychology, 17*, 125–148.

Hudspeth, A.J., & Corey, D. (1977). Sensitivity, polarity and conductance change in the response of vertebrate brain cells to controlled mechanical stimuli. *Proceedings of the National of Academy Sciences USA, 74*, 2407–2411.

Insausti, R., Amaral, D.G., & Cowan, W.M. (1987). The entorhinal cortex of the monkey: II. Cortical afferents. *Journal of Comparative Neurology, 264*, 356–395.

Insel, T.R., Murphy, D.L., & Cohen, R.M. (1983). Obsessive-compulsive disorder: A double-blind trial of clomipramine and clorgyline. *Archives of General Psychiatry, 40*, 605–612.

Izard, C.E. (1971). *The face of emotion.* New York: Appleton-Century-Crofts.

Izard, C.E. (1977). *Human emotions.* New York: Plenum Press.

Izard, C.E. (1981). Differential emotions theory and the facial feedback hypothesis of emotion activation: Comments in Tourajeau and Ellsworth's "The role of facial response in the experience of emotion." *Journal of Personality and Social Psychology, 40*, 350–354.

Izard, C.E. (1982). Comments on emotion and cognition: Can there be a working relationship? In M. Clark & S. Fiske (Eds.), *Affect and cognition* (pp. 229–240). Hillsdale, NJ: Erlbaum.

Izard, C.E. (1993). Four systems for emotion activation: Cognitive and noncognitive processes. *Psychological Review, 100*(1), 68–90.

James, W. (1884). What is emotion? *Mind, 19*, 188–205.

James, W. (1890). *The principles of psychology.* New York: Rinehart & Winston.

Janowsky, D.S., El-Yousef, M.K., & Davis, J.M. (1972). A cholinergic adrenergic hypothesis of mania and depression. *Lancet, 2*, 632–635.

Kandel, E.R., & Hawkins, R.D. (1992, September). The biological basis of learning and individuality. *Scientific American Magazine*, 78–86.

Kaplan, H.I., & Sadock, B.J. (1988). *Synopsis of psychiatry* (5th Ed.). Baltimore: Williams & Wilkins.

Kapp, B.S., & Pascoe, J.P. (1986). Correlation aspects of learning and memory: Vertebrate model systems. In J.L. Martinez & R.P. Kesner (Eds.), *Learning and memory: A biological view* (pp. 399–440). New York: Academic Press.

Kapp, B.S., Pascoe, J.P., & Bixler, M.A. (1984). The amygdala: A neuroanatomical systems approach to its contribution to aversive conditioning. In L.S. Squire & N. Butters (Eds.), *Neuropsychology of memory* (1st ed., pp. 473–488). New York: Guilford Press.

Kellner, C.H. (1993, January 25). Anticonvulsants, ECT, and affective disorders. In *Electroconvulsive therapy and carbamazepine (psychiatry)* (Vol. 22, No. 2, Side A. Audio-Digest Foundation), Glendale, CA.

Kesner, R.P., Walser, R.D., & Winzenried, G. (1988). Central but not basolateral amygdala mediates memory for positive affective experiences. *Behavioral Brain Research, 33*, 189–195.

Kintsch, W. (1970). *Learning, memory and conceptual processes.* New York: Wiley.

Klinger, E., & Cox, W.M. (1987–1988). Dimensions of thought flow in everyday life. *Imagination, Cognition and Personality, 7*, 105–128.

Kluft, R.P. (1984). Treatment of multiple personality disorder: A study of 33 cases. *Psychiatric Clinics of North America, 7*, 9–29.

Kluft, R.P. (1985). Making the diagnosis of multiple personality disorder (MPD). In F.F. Flach (Ed.), *Directions in psychiatry*, New York: Hatherleigh, 5(23): 1–10.

Kohonen, T. (1977). *Associative memory.* Berlin: Springer-Verlag.

Kosslyn, S.M. (1987). Seeing and imagining in the cerebral hemispheres. *Psychological Review, 94*, 148–175.

Kosslyn, S.M. (1988). Aspects of a cognitive neuroscience of imagery. *Science, 240*, 1621–1626.

Kraepelin, E. (1976). *Manic–depressive insanity and paranoia* (R.M. Barclay, Trans.). Edited by G.M. Robertson. Edinburgh: E. and S. Livingstone, 1921. Reprinted New York: Arno Press. Original published in 1921.)

Kuiper, N.A., & Derry, P.A. (1982). Depressed and nondepressed content self-reference in mild depressives. *Journal of Personality, 50*, 67–80.

Lane, H. (1984). *When the mind hears.* New York: Random House.

LeDoux, J.E. (1986). Sensory systems and emotion. *Integrative Psychiatry, 4*, 237–248.

LeDoux, J.E. (1990). Information flow from sensation to emotion: Plasticity in the neural computation of stimulus value. In M. Gabriel & J. Moore (Eds.), *Learning and computational neuroscience: Foundations of adaptive networks* (pp. 3–51). Cambridge, MA: Bradford Books/MIT Press.

LeDoux, J.E., Iwata, J., Cicchetti, P., & Reis, D.J. (1988). Different projections of the central amygdaloid nucleus mediate autonomic and behavioral correlates of conditioned fear. *Journal of Neuroscience, 8*, 2517–2529.

Leventhal, H. (1984). A perceptual motor theory of emotion. In K.R. Scherer and P. Ehman (Eds.), *Approaches to emotion* (pp. 271–291). Hillsdale, NJ: Erlbaum.

Llinas, R. (1990). Intrinsic electrical properties of nerve cells and their role in network oscillation. In E. Kandel, T. Sejnowski, C. Stevens, & J. Watson (Eds.), *Cold Spring Harbor Symposia on Quantitative Biology: The Brain* (Vol. 55, pp. 933–938). New York: Cold Spring Harbor Press.

Lloyd, G.G., & Lishman, W.A. (1975). Effect of depression on the speed of recall of pleasant and unpleasant experiences. *Phychological Medicine, 5*, 173–180.

Ludwig, A.M., Brandsma, J.M., Wilber, C.B., Bendfeldt, F., & Jameson, H. (1972). The objective study of a multiple personality. *Archives of General Psychiatry, 26*, 298–310.

Marcos, L.R., & Trujillo, M. (1978). The sodium amytal interview as a therapeutic modality. *Current Psychiatric Therapies, 18*, 129–136.

Mayes, A.R. (1988). *Human organic memory disorders.* Cambridge, UK: Cambridge University Press.

Mayes, A.R., Meudell, P.R., & Pickering, A.D. (1985). Is organic amnesia caused by a selective deficit in remembering contextual information? *Cortex, 21*, 313–324.

McCarthy, R.A., & Warrington, E.K. (1988). Evidence for modality-specific meaning systems in the brain. *Nature, 334*, 428–430.

McClelland, J.L., & Rumelhart, D.E. (1986). Amnesia and distributed memory. In J.L. McClelland & D.E. Rumelhart (Eds.), *Parallel distributed processing: Explorations in the microstructure of cognition* (pp. 503–527). Cambridge: MIT Press.

McDougall, W. (1910). *An introduction to social psychology* (3rd ed.). Boston: Luce.

McGeoch, J.A. (1932). Forgetting and the law of disuse. *Psychological Review, 39*, 352–370.

McGlashan, T.H. (1983). The borderline syndrome: II. Is it a variant of schizophrenia or affective disorder? *Archives of General Psychiatry, 40*, 1319–1323.

McNaughton, B.L., Douglas, R.M., & Goddard, G.V. (1978). Synaptic enhancement in fascia dentata: Cooperativity among coactive afferents. *Brain Research, 157*, 277–293.

Milestone, S.F. (1993). Implications of affect theory for the practice of cognitive therapy. *Psychiatric Annals, 23*(10), 577–583.

Milner, B. (1970). Memory and the medial temporal regions of the brain. In K.H. Pribram & D.E. Broadbent (Eds.), *Biology of memory* (pp. 29–50). New York: Academic Press.

Milner, B., Corkin, S., & Teuber, H.L. (1968). Further analysis of the hippocampal amnesia syndrome: 14-year follow-up study of H.M. *Neuropsychologia, 6*, 215–234.

Mishkin, M. (1978). Memory in monkeys severely impaired by combined but not by separate removal of amygdala and hippocampus. *Nature, 273*, 297–298.

Mishkin, M., & Appenzeller, T. (1987, June). The anatomy of memory. *Scientific American Magazine*, 88–102.

Moscovitch, M. (1984). The sufficient conditions for demonstrating preserved memory in amnesia: A task analysis. In L.R. Squire & N. Butters (Eds.), *Neuropsychology of memory* (1st ed., pp. 104–114). New York: Guilford Press.

Murphy, D.L., & Beigel, A. (1974). Depression, elation, and lithium carbonate responses in manic patient subgroups. *Archives of General Psychiatry, 31*, 643–648.

Murphy, D.L., Campbell, I., & Costa, J.L. (1978). Current status of the indoleamine hypothesis of the affective disorders. In M.A. Lipton, A. DiMascio, & K.F. Killan (Eds.), *Psychopharmacology: A generation of progress.* New York: Raven Press.

Murphy, G. (1923). Types of word-association in dementia praecox, manic–depressives, and normal persons. *American Journal of Psychiatry, 79*, 539–571.

Naples, M., & Hackett, T.P. (1978). The amytal interview: History and current uses. *Psychosomatics, 19*, 98–105.

Nathanson, D.L. (1993). About emotion. *Psychiatric Annals, 23*(10), 543–555.

Nathanson, D.L., & Pfrommer, J.M. (1993). Affect theory and psychopharmacology. *Psychiatric Annals, 23*(10), 584–593.

Newcombe, F., Young, A., & DeHaan, E.H.F. (1989). Prosopagnosia and object agnosia without covert recognition. *Neuropsychologia, 27*, 179–191.

Newman, L., & Hirt, J. (1983). The psychoanalytic theory of depression symptoms as a function of aggressive wishes and level of field articulation. *Journal of Abnormal Psychology, 92*, 42–48.

Olds, J. (1956, October). Pleasure centers in the brain. *Scientific American Magazine*, 105–116.

Olds, J., & Milner, P. (1954). Positive reinforcement produced by electrical stimulation of septal area and other regions of rat brain. *Journal of Comparative and Physiological Psychology, 47*, 419–427.

Ornstein, R. (1986). *The psychology of consciousness.* New York: Penguin Books.

Ornstein, R. (1991). *The evolution of consciousness.* New York: Prentice-Hall.

Ornstein, R., & Thompson, R.F. (1986). *The amazing brain.* Boston: Houghton Mifflin.

Overton, D.A. (1964). State-dependent or "dissociated" learning produced by pentobarbital. *Journal of Comparative and Physiological Psychology, 57*, 3–12.

Paillard, J., Michel, F., & Stelmach, G. (1983). Localization without content: A tactile analogue of "blind sight." *Archives of Neurology, 40*, 548–551.

Paivio, A. (1986). *Mental representations: A dual coding approach.* Oxford: Oxford University Press.

Palm, G. (1980). On associative memory. *Biological Cybernetics, 36*, 19–31.

Papanicolaou, A.C. (1989). *Emotion: A reconsideration of the somatic theory.* New York: Gordon & Breach.

Pavlov, I.P. (1927). *Conditioned reflexes.* (G.V. Anrep, Trans.). New York: Oxford University Press.

Peterson, C., & Seligman, M. (1984). Causal explanations as a risk factor for depression: Theory and evidence. *Psychological Review, 91*, 347–375.

Plutchik, R. (1980). *Emotion: A psychoevolutionary synthesis.* New York: Harper & Row.

Pope, H.G., Jonas, J.M., Hudson, J.I., Cohen, B.M., & Gunderson, J.G. (1983). The validity of DSM-III borderline personality disorder: A phenomenologic, family history treatment response, and long-term follow-up study. *Archives of General Psychiatry, 40*, 23–30.

Post, R.M. (1993, January 11). The course of bipolar affective disorder: Implications for treatment. In *Mesoridazine: The course of bipolar disorder (psychiatry)* (Vol. 2, No. 1, Sides A and B), Audio-Digest Foundation.

Putnam, F.W. (1986). The scientific investigation of multiple personality disorder. In J.M. Quen (Ed.), *Split minds/split brains* (pp. 109–125). New York: New York University Press.

Putnam, F.W. (1989). *Diagnosis and treatment of multiple personality disorder.* New York: Guilford Press.

Putnam, F.W., Guroff, J.J., Silberman, E.K., Barban, L., & Post, R.M. (1986). The clinical phenomenology of multiple personality disorder: A review of 100 recent cases. *Journal of Clinical Psychiatry, 47,* 285–293.

Racine, R.J., Milgram, N.W., & Hafner, S., Long-term potentiation phenomena in the rat limbic forebrain. *Brain Research, 260,* 217–231.

Rapaport, D. (1971). *Emotions and memory.* New York: International Universities Press.

Rapoport, J.L. (1989, March). The biology of obsessions and compulsions. *Scientific American Magazine,* 82–89.

Restak, R.M. (1984). *The brain.* New York: Bantam Books.

Restak, R.M. (1988). *The mind.* New York: Bantam Books.

Reynolds, C.F., & Kupfer, D.J. (1988). Sleep in depression. In R.L. Williams, I. Karacan, & C.A. Moore (Eds.), *Sleep disorders: Diagnosis and treatment* (2nd ed., pp. 147–164). New York: Wiley.

Ribot, T. (1910). *The diseases of personality.* Chicago: Kegan Paul, Trench, Trubner.

Richardson-Klavehn, A., & Bjork, R.A. (1988). Measures of memory. *Annual Review of Psychology, 39,* 475–543.

Rizley, R., & Rescorla, R. (1972). Associations in second-order conditioning and sensory preconditioning. *Journal of Comparative and Physiological Psychology, 81,* 1–11.

Rolls, E.T. (1990). Functions of neuronal networks in the hippocampus and of backprojections in the cerebral cortex in memory. In J.L. McGaugh, N.M. Weinberger, & G. Lynch (eds.), *Brain organization and memory: Cells, systems and circuits* (pp. 184–210). New York: Oxford University Press.

Rosenblatt, F. (1961). *Principles of neurodynamics: Perceptrons and the theory of brain mechanisms.* Washington, DC: Spartan Books.

Rosenfield, I. (1992). *The strange, familiar and forgotten: An anatomy of consciousness.* New York: Knopf.

Rosenthal, N.E., Rosenthal, L.N., Stallone, F., Dunner, D.L., & Fieve, R.R. (1980). Toward the validation of RDC schizoaffective disorder. *Archives of General Psychiatry, 37,* 804–810.

Ross, C.A. (1989). *Multiple personality disorder: Diagnosis, clinical features, and treatment.* New York: Wiley.

Ross, C.A., Norton, G.R., & Wozney, K. (1989). Multiple personality disorder: An analysis of 236 cases. *Canadian Journal of Psychiatry, 34*(5), 413–418.

Routtenberg, A. (1978, November). The reward system of the brain. *Scientific American Magazine,* 75–87.

Ruedrich, S.L., Chu, C.-C., & Wadle, C.V. (1985). The amytal interview in the treatment of psychogenic amnesia. *Hospital and Community Psychiatry, 36,* 1045–1046.

Russell, W.R., & Nathan, P.W. (1946). Traumatic amnesia. *Brain, 68,* 280–300.

Santa, J.L., & Lamwers, L.A. (1974). Encoding specificity: Fact or artifact? *Journal of Verbal Learning and Verbal Behavior, 13,* 412–423.

Schachter, S., & Singer, J.F. (1962). Cognitive, social and physiological determinants of emotional state. *Psychological Review, 69,* 337, 379–399.

Schacter, D.L. (1987). Implicit memory: History and current status. *Journal of Experimental Psychology: Learning, Memory and Cognition, 13,* 501–518.

Schacter, D.L. (1989). On the relation between memory and consciousness: Dissociable interactions and conscious experience. In H.L. Roediger & F.I.M. Craik (Eds.), *Varieties of memory and consciousness* (pp. 355–389). Hillsdale, NJ: Erlbaum.

Schacter, D.L. (1990). Toward a cognitive neuropsychology of awareness: Implicit knowledge and anosognosia. *Journal of Clinical and Experimental Neuropsychology, 12,* 155–178.

Schacter, D.L., Harbluk, J.L., & McLachlan, D.R. (1984). Retrieval without recollection: An experimental analysis of source amnesia. *Journal of Verbal Learning and Verbal Behavior, 23,* 593–611.

Schank, R.C. (1982). *Dynamic memory: A theory of reminding and learning in computers and people.* New York: Cambridge University Press.

Schank, R.C., & Abelson, R.P. (1977). *Scripts, plans, goals and understanding: An inquiry into human knowledge structures.* Hillsdale, NJ: Erlbaum.

Scherer, K.R. (1988). Cognitive antecedents of emotion. In V. Hamilton, G.H. Bower, & N.H. Frijda (Eds.), *Cognitive perspectives on emotion and motivation* (pp. 89–126). Dordrecht, The Netherlands: Martinus Nijhoff.

Schildkraut, J.J. (1965). The catecholamine hypothesis of affective disorders: A review of supporting evidence. *American Journal of Psychiatry, 122,* 509–522.

Scoville, W.B., & Milner, B. (1957). Loss of recent memory after bilateral hippocampal lesions. *Journal of Neurology, Neurosurgery and Psychiatry, 20,* 11–12.

Segal, S., & Fusella, V. (1970). Influence of imaged pictures and sounds on detection of visual and auditory signals. *Journal of Experimental Psychology, 83,* 458–464.

Shimamura, A.P., & Squire, L.R. (1987). A neuropsychological study of fact learning and source amnesia. *Journal of Experimental Psychology: Learning, Memory and Cognition, 13,* 464–474.

Small, J.G., Klapper, M.H., Kellams, J.J., Miller, M.J., Milstein, V., Sharpley, P.H., & Small, I.F. (1988). Electroconvulsive treatment compared with lithium in the management of manic states. *Archives of General Psychiatry, 45,* 727–732.

Smith, C.A., & Ellsworth, P.C. (1985). Patterns of cognitive appraisal in emotion. *Journal of Personality and Social Psychology, 48,* 813–838.

Solomon, R. (1983). The use of the MMPI with multiple personality patients. *Psychological Reports, 53,* 1004–1006.

Spanos, N.P., Weekes, J.R., & Bertrand, L.D. (1985). Multiple personality: A social psychological perspective. *Journal of Abnormal Psychology, 94,* 362–376.

Squire, L.R. (1986). Mechanisms of memory. *Science, 232,* 1612–1619.

Squire, L.R. (1987a). *Memory and brain.* New York: Oxford University Press.

Squire, L.R. (1987b). Complex connections involved in memory functions. In J. Byrne & W.O. Berry (Eds.), *Neural models of plasticity: Theoretical and empirical approaches.* Orlando, FL.: Academic Press.

Squire, L.R. (1992). Memory and the hippocampus: A synthesis from findings with rats, monkeys and humans. *Psychological Review, 99*(2), 195–231.

Squire, L.R., Shimamura, A.P., & Amaral, D.G. (1989). Memory and the hippocampus. In J. Byrne & W. Berry (Eds.), *Neural models of plasticity.* New York: Academic Press.

Squire, L.R., & Zola-Morgan, S. (1988). Memory: Brain systems and behavior. *Trends in Neurosciences, 11,* 170–175.

Squire, L.R., & Zola-Morgan, S. (1991). The medial temporal lobe memory system. *Science, 253,* 1380–1386.

Stanton, P.K., & Sejnowski, T.J. (1989). Associative long-term depression in the hippocampus induced by Hebbian covariance. *Nature, 339,* 215–218.

Stone, A.M. (1993). Trauma and affect: Applying the language of affect theory to the phenomena of traumatic stress. *Psychiatric Annals, 23*(10), 567–576.

"Stranger in the Mirror" (1993, December). *Nova.* New York: Public Broadcasting Service.

Taylor, M.A., & Abrams, R. (1977). Catatonia: Prevalence and importance in the manic phase of manic–depressive illness. *Archives of General Psychiatry, 34,* 1223–1225.

Thompson, J. (1941). Development of facial expression of emotion in blind and seeing children. *Archives of Psychology, 37*(264).

Thorndike, E.L. (1903). *Educational psychology.* New York: Lemcke & Buechner.

Thorndike, E.L., & Woodworth, R.S. (1901). The influence of improvement in one mental function upon the efficiency of other functions. *Psychological Review, 8,* 247–261, 384–395, 553–564.

Tomkins, S.S. (1962). *Affect, imagery, consciousness: Vol. I. The positive affects.* New York: Springer.

Tomkins, S.S. (1963). *Affect, imagery, consciousness. Vol. II: The negative affects.* New York: Springer.

Tranel, D., & Damasio, A.R. (1985). Knowledge without awareness: An autonomic index of facial recognition by prosopagnosics. *Science, 228,* 1453–1454.

Tulving, E. (1972). Episodic and semantic memory. In E. Tulving & W. Donaldson (Eds.), *The organization of memory* (pp. 382–404). New York: Academic Press.

Tulving, E. (1983). *Elements of episodic memory.* New York: Oxford University Press.

Tulving, E. (1985). How many memory systems are there? *American Psychologist, 40,* 385–398.

Tulving, E. (1987). Multiple memory systems and consciousness. *Human Neurobiology, 6,* 67–80.

Tulving, E. (1989). Memory, performance, knowledge and experience. *European Journal of Cognitive Psychology, 1,* 3–26.

Tulving, E., Schacter, D.L., & Stark, H.A. (1982). Priming effects in word-fragment completion are independent of recognition memory. *Journal of Experimental Psychology: Learning, Memory and Cognition, 8,* 336–342.

Tulving, E., & Thomson, D.M. (1973). Encoding specificity and retrieval processes in episodic memory. *Psychological Review, 80,* 353–373.

Turner, S.M., Jacob, R.G., Beidel, D.C., & Himmelhoch, J. (1985). Fluoxetine treatment of obsessive–compulsive disorder. *Journal of Clinical Psychopharmacology, 5,* 207–212.

Van Hoesen, G.W. (1982). The parahippocampal gyrus. New observations regarding its cortical connections in the monkey. *Trends in Neurosciences, 5,* 345–350.

von der Malsburg, C. (1990). A neural architecture for the representation of scenes. In J.L. McGaugh, N.M. Weinberger, & G. Lynch (Eds.), *Brain organization and memory: Cells, systems and circuits* (pp. 356–372). New York: Oxford University Press.

Warrington, E.K., & Weiskrantz, L. (1974). The effect of prior learning on subsequent retention in amnesic patients. *Neuropsychologia, 12,* 419–428.

Warrington, E.K., & McCarthy, R.A. (1987). Categories of knowledge: Further fractionations and an attempted integration. *Brain, 110,* 1273–1296.

Watkins, M.J., & Gardiner, J.M. (1979). An appreciation of generate–recognize theory of recall. *Journal of Verbal Learning and Verbal Behavior, 18,* 687–704.

Weiner, B. (1985). An attributional theory of achievement, motivation and emotion. *Psychological Review, 92,* 548–573.

Weingartner, H., Miller, H., & Murphy, D.L. (1977). Mood-state–dependent retrieval of verbal associations. *Journal of Abnormal Psychology, 86,* 276–284.

Weiskrantz, L. (1956). Behavioral changes associated with ablation of the amygdaloid complex in monkeys. *Journal of Comparative and Physiological Psychology, 49,* 381–391.

Weissman, M.M. (1978). Psychotherapy and its relevance to the pharmacotherapy of affective disorders: From ideology to evidence. In M.A. Lipton, A. DiMascio, & K.F. Killam (Eds.), *Psychopharmacology: A generation of progress* (pp. 1313–1321). New York: Raven Press.

Wickelgren, W.A. (1977). *Learning and memory.* Englewood Cliffs, NJ: Prentice-Hall.

Wickelgren, W.A. (1979). Chunking and consolidation. *Psychological Review, 86,* 44–60.

Williams, J.M.G., & Broadbent, D.E. (1986). Autobiographical memory in suicide attempters. *Journal of Abnormal Psychology, 95,* 145–149.

Williams, J.M.G., Watts, F.N., Macleod, C., & Mathews, A. (1988). *Cognitive psychology and emotional disorders.* Chichester, UK: Wiley.

Willshaw, D.J., Buneman, O.P., & Longuet-Higgins, H.C. (1969). Non-holographic associative memory. *Nature, 222,* 960–962.

Winokur, G., Clayton, P.J., & Reich, T. (1969). *Manic–depressive illness.* St.Louis: C.V. Mosby.

Wolpe, J. (1958). *Psychotherapy by reciprocal inhibition.* Stanford, CA: Stanford University Press.

Worchel, S., & Shebilske, W. (1986). *Psychology: Principles and applications* (2nd ed.). Englewood Cliffs, NJ: Prentice-Hall.

Zola-Morgan, S., & Squire, L.R. (1990a). The primate hippocampal formation: Evidence for a time-limited role in memory storage. *Science, 250,* 288–290.

Zola-Morgan, S., & Squire, L.R. (1990b). The neuropsychology of memory: Parallel findings from humans and nonhuman primates. *Annals of the New York Academy of Science, 608,* 434–456.

Zola-Morgan, S., Squire, L.R., Alvarez-Royo, P., & Clower, R.P. (1991). Independence of memory functions and emotional behavior: Separate contributions of the hippocampal formation and the amygdala. *Hippocampus, 1,* 207–220.

Zola-Morgan, S., Squire, L.R., Amaral, D.G., & Suzuki, W. (1989). Lesions of perirhinal and parahippocampal cortex that spare the amygdala and hippocampal formation produce severe memory impairment. *Journal of Neuroscience, 9,* 4355–4370.

Index